D1287002

Medicine & Society
In America

Medicine & Society In America

Advisory Editor

Charles E. Rosenberg
Professor of History
University of Pennsylvania

MEDICINE IN VIRGINIA

in the

SEVENTEENTH CENTURY

by

WYNDHAM B. BLANTON, M. D.

ARNO PRESS & THE NEW YORK TIMES

New York   1972

Reprint Edition 1972 by Arno Press Inc.

Reprinted from a copy in
The Duke University Medical Center Library

LC# 77-180556
ISBN 0-405-03936-0

Medicine and Society in America
ISBN for complete set: 0-405-03930-1
See last pages of this volume for titles.

Manufactured in the United States of America

MEDICINE IN VIRGINIA

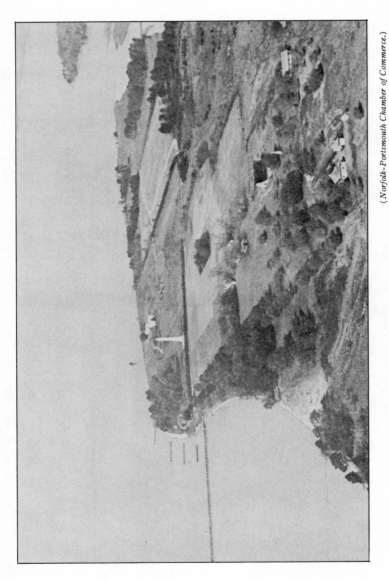

(*Norfolk-Portsmouth Chamber of Commerce.*)

The site of Jamestown, photographed from the air.

MEDICINE IN VIRGINIA

in the

SEVENTEENTH CENTURY

by

WYNDHAM B. BLANTON, M. D.

PUBLISHERS

THE WILLIAM BYRD PRESS, INC.

RICHMOND

FOREWORD

During his incumbency as President of the Medical Society of Virginia in 1926-27 Dr. J. W. Preston of Roanoke, realizing the need for a history of Virginia medicine, secured the appointment of an historical committee. Dr. Wyndham B. Blanton of Richmond, Dr. Frederick Rinker of Norfolk, and Dr. Beverley R. Tucker of Richmond constituted the committee, with Dr. Blanton as chairman.

It was early decided that the work was not to consist merely of a brief biographical notice of individual physicians but was to be a moving word picture of Virginia medical development, with the physician playing his part in the foreground. It was thought best to divide the work into three periods and attempt to make it as adequate as possible regardless of how many volumes were required or how much time it took.

The present volume embraces the progress of medicine in that period of Virginia history from 1607 to 1700. Subsequent volumes will cover the Eighteenth and Nineteenth Centuries.

Your present committee asks that the Society will be both generous and patient in its attitude toward the completion of this work, in order that posterity may have in hand a record of Virginia's contribution to the progress of medicine in this country, both in institutions and in physicians, for we believe that no state has more right to be proud of its medical achievements. The highest incentive toward the medical de-

[ix]

velopment of Virginia in the future is the inspiration of the past, and the deeds which have been wrought and the lives that have been in labor spent will form a part of a living force as well as give the heritage of a glorious tradition.

To accomplish the requirements of a subject so vast and yet so comprehensive, the co-operation of the members of the Society is essential.

Your committee wishes to take this occasion to thank the Society for its aid and indulgence and hopes that the reception of this first volume will merit a continuation of its support and generosity, without which nothing really worth while can be accomplished.

Mrs. Ralph T. Catterall has ably collaborated with the author in the research for this volume. Her keen interest and efficiency have been of great service. We are indebted to Dr. Joseph L. Miller for a number of illustrations from his fine collection of rare Seventeenth Century books.

BEVERLY RANDOLPH TUCKER.

TABLE OF CONTENTS

LIST OF ILLUSTRATIONS

INTRODUCTION

By the beginning of the Seventeenth Century anatomy was on a sound basis, and the average doctor knew pretty well the coarse structures of the human body. Physiology had made a good start, and medicine was beginning to understand how the human machine worked. The other fundamental branches were unknown. Obstetrics was in the hands of midwives. Although in the treatment of disease the profession had at its disposal a large assortment of empirical remedies, much of its therapy was more harmful than good. To its skirts still clung much of ancient superstition and many ponderous theories of disease. There was no real knowledge of what disease was, of its location in the body, or of its causes. Happily, the advance of medical knowledge since that time has been phenomenal, bridging the great hiatus that separates an art from a science.

No small part of this recent progress has been made in America, and American medicine has come to mean something distinctive. For three centuries medicine has been in the making on this continent, and while our greatest advance has come in the last generation there were factors at work in the earlier centuries which have to be considered in any true account of the development of the science in this country.

Early colonial medicine was not creative or epoch-making; nor did it altogether reflect continental medicine. It assumed, by the exigencies of the time, features which were peculiarly indigenous. Without cities, hospitals, professional contacts, books or instruments the early colonial doctor acquired a resourcefulness, independence of action, courage and ingenuity bred only in the school of real necessity.

Fortune planted the first English colony in America on the shores of Virginia. Her domain early became the most extensive of all the colonies. The enterprise of her citizens rapidly raised her to a position of leadership among her neighbors. Interest in things Virginian has hitherto centered elsewhere than in medicine, the story of which has lain fossilized in the early county records, colonial documents and casual writings of contemporary authors. Medicine in the Seventeenth Century in Virginia was much as it was in the other colonies. It was not a productive but a fallow time, out of which some very real contributions flowered during the succeeding centuries. The first Caesarian section and the first oophorectomy in America were performed by a pioneer Virginia doctor. Likewise to Virginia belongs priority on this continent in operations for cleft palate and club foot, in the use of the plaster cast in the treatment of tuberculosis of the spine, and of metallic sutures in vesicovaginal repair. A Virginian promulgated the theory of evolution before Darwin, and another described typhoid fever thirteen years before Louis. Still another advocated the use of steam in the disinfection of infected ships. The first American pharmacopeia, the first autopsy, the first hospital, the first insane asylum on this continent were Virginia achievements, and the earliest bill governing medical practice was drawn by the Virginia Assembly; while the first American college to teach comparative anatomy, to institute the ten month medical course, and to take a stand for adequate premedical education was the University of Virginia.

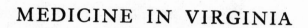

MEDICINE IN VIRGINIA

MEDICINE IN VIRGINIA

CHAPTER I

MEDICINE UNDER THE LONDON COMPANY
1607–1624

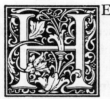ENRY KENTON was an English surgeon attached to the fleet of Captain Bartholomew Gilbert. This fleet was exploring Virginia waters in 1603, the year Queen Elizabeth died. While in the "Chesepian Bay in the country of Virginia" a landing party of five went ashore, among them the surgeon. An Indian ambush, a sudden sally, and the little party perished to a man.[1] Years came and went, and other adventurous doctors found their way to Virginia, but the forgotten ship-surgeon, Henry Kenton, was the first English physician to land upon the American continent and the first to lose his life in line of duty. That was one of the incidents of exploration.

Colonization followed feebly in the wake of a century of daring exploration. For eighteen years—until 1624, when James I assumed entire control of the colony—affairs in Virginia were managed by the London Company under powers delegated to it in three separate royal charters. The Company was a private enterprise, made up of distinguished personages, and like the East India Company and the Plymouth

---

[1]Brown: Genesis of the U. S., v. 1, p. 27.

Company it made possible the great English trading and colonization projects of the Seventeen Century. Its interests in Virginia were on the whole lofty. There was no intentional exploitation of the colony. In the minds of those far-seeing Englishmen new world colonization was intimately connected with the very life of the nation—a nation already dependent upon foreign trade for the maintenance of many of its basic industries. A colony on the shores of Virginia meant a trade the mother country could always control, in wood to build ships and operate furnaces, in drugs, wines, silk, grain, possibly in precious ores. It meant a place to send England's overflow population. To some, perhaps, it meant an asylum for criminals; to others, an opportunity to educate and christianize the heathen Indian. The serious purpose behind the Company is reflected in the type of medical men connected with it and in the health measures which it repeatedly adopted.

Among the English physicians who were interested in Virginia colonization or were members of the Company none was more distinguished than Dr. Theodore Gulstone, an Oxford graduate, who was censor of the College of Physicians and one of its real benefactors. He owned six shares of land in Virginia and was responsible for the choice of one of her physicians-general. Peter Turner was also a subscriber in the Company. He was physician to Sir Walter Raleigh, and in 1606 submitted a report on the decline of Raleigh's health in the tower. Another subscriber was Leonard Poe, one of the King's physicians, who attended

Salisbury in his last illness.   Still another was Thomas Winston, professor of physic at Gresham College.   The list also includes John Woodall, author of *The Chirurgion's Mate,* who was interested in sending cattle to Virginia because he considered milk essential to the colony; Thomas Hood, who sailed around the world with Drake; Thomas Lodge, Francis Anthony, Anthony Hinton, William Turner, and Peter Maunsell.[2]

That these men were mindful of the health of the colony is to be seen in the very specific directions as to its location, which they gave the first planters, in the type of medical men they sponsored, in the number of apothecaries they sent over, in their specifications for hospitals, and in other important measures.

Four years after the death of Henry Kenton the English voyages of exploration in the new world developed into something more concrete.   In May 1607 a small group of colonists, sent out by the London Company, sailed forty miles up the James River, landed on an island,* and named their settlement James City.   From that moment life was busy, anxious and uncertain.   There were hazards on all sides.   Grave danger lay in the explorations of Smith and Newport, in the planting of new industries such as the glass and iron works, in the administration of the government with its bickerings and jealousies, charges and counter-

---

[2]Brown: Genesis of the U. S., v. 1, pp. 209-228; v. 2, appendix.
*A marsh and not the present stream is said to have separated the colony from the mainland.

charges.   Worse than these were the silent, terrifying
ravages of disease.   The English had reckoned more with
wounds and injuries than with sickness, and no physician was
included among the first planters.   Two "chirurgeons" were
counted a liberal allowance of medical aid.

One of the chirurgeons was Will Wilkinson.   We have
no record of him other than the inclusion of his name in the
list of planters.[3]   He was classed with "Will Garret the
Brick layer" and "Tho: Cowper the Barber" and was man-
ifestly not a "gentleman."   The inclusion of a barber in the
personnel of the adventurers at a time when there was no
very sharp distinction between surgery and barbering leads
us to believe that the early Virginia chirurgeons were relieved of this distasteful sideline of their profession.   The
term "barber-surgeon" does not appear in the Virginia records, and it is to be inferred that the cleft between the two
professions was real and permanent in the colony.

The gentleman chirurgeon was Thomas Wotton.[4] Wotton
was a good name in England.   Edward Wotton, M. D.
(1494-1555), studied at Padua, had been King's physician
in the time of Henry VIII, and had written a famous work
on natural history.   Henry Wotton, M. D., his son, was a
distinguished fellow of the Royal College of Physicians, and
is last heard of in 1582, when he was a candidate for physician to St. Bartholomew's Hospital.   Thomas Wotton may
have been his son.   In any event he had his hands full at

---

[3]Smith: General History of Virginia, p. 390.
[4]Ibid.

Jamestown those first eight months, when he and Wilkinson were the entire medical force. He should have exerted his influence in the selection of a site for the colony, but his voice was either not heeded or not raised. The Company's instructions, "neither must you plant in a low or moist place because it will prove unhealthful," were entirely disregarded.

Captain John Smith praised the service rendered by Wotton in the summer of 1607. Perhaps he had reason for it in his own recovery, for he wrote, "Smith newly recovered, Martin and Ratcliffe was by his care preserved and relieved, and the most of the souldiers recovered, with the skillful diligence of Mr. Thomas Wotton our Chirurgion generall."[5] President Wingfield, on the other hand, explained that he has made an enemy of "Thomas Wootton, the surieon, because I would not subscribe to a Warrant to the Treasurer of Virginia, to deliver him money to furnish him with druggs and other necessaryes; & because I disallowed his living in the pinnasse, haveing many of our men lyeing sick & wounded in our towne, to whose dressings by that meanes he slacked his attendance."[6] Evidently the chirurgeon was a cautious man. It was undoubtedly safer to live on shipboard and avoid the hazard of Indian tomahawks and arrows at Jamestown.

What happened to Wotton after two years in the colony is uncertain. Smith says he was not there in 1609. In 1635 Sir William Curteen made a voyage to the East Indies,

---

[5]Smith: General History of Virginia, p. 392.
[6]Wingfield: Discourse of Virginia, p. 41.

and with him went one Thomas Wotton, "Barber-Cirur-geon," whose will, made at the time of the voyage, was proved in England, April 28, 1638.[7] This may very probably have been our sometime Virginia Chirurgeon General.

The first supply of 120 settlers reached the colony in January 1608, to find only forty of the original planters remaining. With this supply came medical reinforcements in the persons of Dr. Walter Russell, physician, Post Ginnat, chirurgeon, and two apothecaries, Thomas Field and John Harford.[8]

Walter Russell was the first physician, as distinguished from the chirurgeon, to come to this country. He had something of Captain Smith's adventurous spirit and was included in the company that explored Chesapeake Bay, June 1608. The party named some of their newly discovered islands after the "doctor of physicke" and spent "the next day searching those inhabitable Isles (which we called Russell's Isles) to provide fresh water."[9] It was on this trip that Dr. Russell rendered much appreciated service to Captain Smith: "But it chanced, the Captaine taking a fish from his sword (not knowing her condition), being much of the fashion of a Thornebacke with a longer taile whereon is a most poysoned sting 2 or 3 inches long, which shee strooke an inch and halfe into the wrist of his arme: the which in 4 houres, had so extremely swolne his hand, arme, shoulder,

---

[7]Virginia Magazine of History and Biography. v. 22, p. 25.
[8]Smith: General History of Virginia, pp. 411, 412.
[9]Ibid., pp. 109, 110.

and part of his body, as we all with much sorrow concluded his funerall, & prepared his grave in an Ile hard by (as himselfe appointed) which then wee called Stingeray Ile, after the name of the fish. Yet by the helpe of a precious oile, Doctour Russel applyed, ere night his tormenting paine was so wel asswaged that he eate the fish to his supper; which gave no less joy and content to us, then ease to himselfe. Having neither Surgeon nor surgerie but that preservative oile we presently set saile for James Towne."[10] Stingray Point is still to be found on the maps of Virginia. Dr. Walter Russell and Amos Todkill were credited by Smith with the authorship of this account, which thus forms a part of the first literary effort of an American physician.

We hear nothing further of Post Ginnat or the two apothecaries; but another interesting chirurgeon, first mentioned in 1608, had come in either with the first planters or the first supply. Anthony Bagnall[11] supplanted Dr. Russell on the second expedition up the bay, and though he did not save Smith's life he excited his admiration as a good shot. "Somewhere on the Pauamunkee," it is recorded, "an hundred and forty-eight foules the President, Anthony Bagnall, and Serjeant Pising did kill at three shots."[12] On one of their encounters with the Indians "none were hurt only Anthony Bagnall was shot in his Hat and another in his sleeve."[13] During the same expedition, when they discovered

---

[10]Smith: General History of Virginia, p. 114.
[11]Ibid., p. 421.
[12]Ibid., p. 449.
[13]Ibid., p. 432.

that "there lay a savage as dead, shot in the knee . . . we had him to our boat where our chirurgian who went with us to cure our Captaine's hurt of the stingray so dressed this Salvage that within an hour he looked somewhat chearfully and did eate and speake."[14]   Why Captain Smith should have preferred the chirurgeon, Bagnall, to the physician, Russell, on his second expedition is not stated.   Possibly the stingray wound, which he still had, presented surgical rather than medical problems.

Smith, himself, had a very good idea of medicine, acquired out of a wide experience.   In his *Sea Grammar* he specified the duties and qualifications of the chirurgeon.   He seems also to have practised medicine when the occasion demanded it.   Once an Indian prisoner at Jamestown was almost smothered to death in his dungeon and so "pittiously" burnt that little hope was held out for his recovery.   Smith promised the man's brother to "make him alive again."   This he did by filling the sufferer full of aquavitae and vinegar and putting him before a fire to sleep.   The treatment worked wonders.   In the morning the wounds were dressed, and the prisoner and his brother "went away so well contented, that this was spread among all the Salvages for a miracle, that Captaine Smith could make a man alive that is dead."[15]

Smith's administration was called very cruel by his enemies, but according to his own account "there died not past seven" out of 200 persons during the winter of 1608-09.   In 1609

---

[14]Smith: General History of Virginia, p. 427.
[15]Ibid., p. 470.

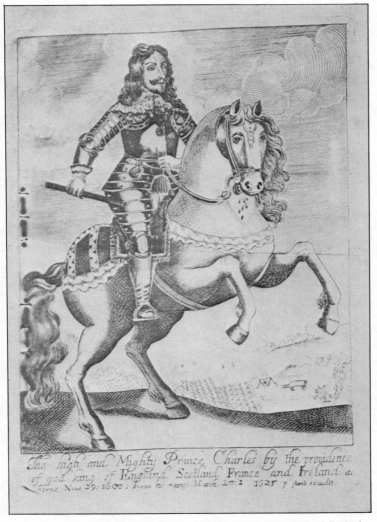

The high and Mighty Prince Charles by the providence
of god king of England Scotland France and Ireland &c
Borne Novē 19: 1600: Began his raigne March 27:2 1625 y Smith excudit

Frontispiece of Woodall's *Surgeon's Mate,* a book often found in
Seventeenth Century Virginia libraries.

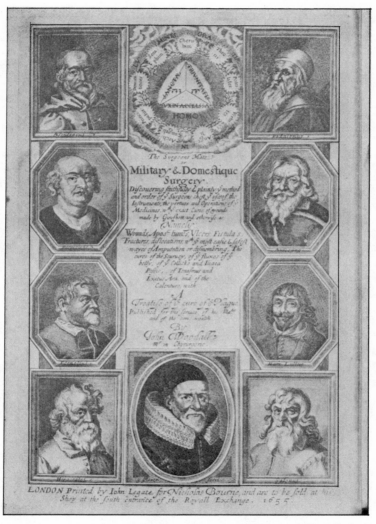

Title page of Woodall's *Surgeon's Mate,* often found in Seventeenth Century Virginia libraries. Woodall's portrait is at the lower center of the page.

he received a severe burn from a gun powder explosion, which necessitated his return to England "because there was neither chirurgeon or chirurgerye in the fort." Evidently he did not care to practise upon himself, although he had acquired a reputation among the Indians in a similar circumstance. The severity of Smith's burn is open to question. It scarcely explains his sudden decision to take to the sea, for the wound would probably have fared better at Jamestown than on shipboard. One suspects that Smith had had his fill of colonial broils, and returned to England with every intention of staying there.

When Lord Delaware came to Virginia in 1610, he brought with him a physician of some parts, Lawrence Bohun, "Doctor in phisick."[16] He is the second physician mentioned in the colonial records as coming to Virginia, and is said to have been "a long time brought up amongst the most learned Surgeons and physitions in the Netherlands."[17]

A letter from the Governor and Council to the London Company, July 7, 1610, gives a vivid picture of widespread sickness and exhausted medicine chests, and describes the physician's diligence during this disastrous period in the colony's history: "Mr. Dr. Boone [Bohun] whose care and industrie for the preservation of our men's lives (assaulted with strange fluxes and agues), we have just cause to commend unto your noble favours; nor let it, I beseech yee, be

---

[16]Brown: Genesis of the U. S., v. 2, p. 830.
[17]Ibid.

passed over as a motion slight and of no moment to furnish us with these things . . . since we have true experience how many men's lives these physicke helpes have preserved since our coming in, God so blessing the practise and diligence of our doctor, whose store has nowe growne thereby to so low an ebb, as we have not above 3 weekes phisicall provisions, if our men continew still thus visited with the sicknesses of the countrie, of the which every season hath his particular infirmities reigning in it, as we have it related unto us by the old inhabitants; and since our owne arrivall, have cause to feare it to be true, who have had 150 at a time much afflicted, and I am perswaded had lost the greatest part of them, if we had not brought these helpes with us."[18]

Sickness and a dwindling medical supply stimulated Bohun to investigate the medicinal properties of the native plants. He must have had talent, boldness and the scientific spirit, and the accounts of Strachey and Smith are at some pains to proclaim his discoveries. He experimented with Sassafras, which grew in abundance about Jamestown and which had so captivated the first planters that they wasted precious hours packing it into the hulls of returning ships. Another plant, called *galbanum mechoacon,* or *rubarbum album,* was used by Dr. Bohun "in cold and moist bodies, for the purginge of Fleame and superfluous matter."[19] Either Strachey or Bohun must have belonged to the Humeral School, which laid great store by the elements—fire, air,

---

[18]Neill: Virginia Company of London, p. 48.
[19]Strachey: Travailes, pp. 31, 32.

earth and water; the qualities—hot, dry, moist and cold; and the humours—blood, phlegm, yellow and black bile. By a curious "permutation and combination" of these components the Humeral pathologist of that day worked out his diagnosis and therapy, for naturally he regarded all disease as a maladjustment of one or the other of them. Dr. Bohun also had great faith in a local product which he called *Terra Alba Virginensis,* an argillaceous earth which was really nothing but a white clay, said to possess absorbent and alexipharmic (poison expelling) properties. It was described as "both aromatical and cordiall, and diapharetick" and was recommended in pestilent and malignant fevers.[20] The inquisitive mind of Bohun led him to investigate the properties of the gums of the local trees. He found that the gum of white poplar and of another tree very much like it was clear and odoriferous and not unlike turpentine. He at once perceived that it would make a good balsam and so applied it. The result was thoroughly satisfactory, and it was said to "heale any green wound." Another interesting tree on Jamestown Island was "small of leaves, armes, and fruict, like the mirtle tree." The fruit tasted like the myrtle, but was found to be much more "bynding." "These trees growe in great plentie, round about a standing pond of fresh water in the middle of the island, the pill or rind whereof is of a great force against inveterate dissentericall fluxes." Dr. Bohun was determined to experiment with this anti-

---

[20]Strachey: Travailes, pp. 31, 32.

dysenteric and used it extensively in the epidemic of diarrheas then raging. Moreover, he "wisheth all such phisitians as shall goe thither to make use thereof."[21]

Dr. Bohun's experiments were brought to an untimely close by the fact that his most distinguished patient, Lord Delaware, had a disease (scurvy) which would yield only to the citrous fruits of the West Indies. The Governor, sick, and tired of Virginia, set sail in 1611, taking Bohun with him. "On the 28th of March, he shipped himself, with Dr. Bohun . . . for Mevis, in the West Indies, at that time famous for wholesome Baths. But . . . they were obliged to shape their course to the Western-Islands; where his Lordship met with much Relief from Oranges & Lemons, a sovereign Remedy for that Disorder."[22]

Whether or not Dr. Bohun came back to Virginia is uncertain. In 1612 he was one of the new adventurers listed under the third charter, and prior to February 2, 1620, with "James Swifte esquire," he was granted patents for the transportation to Virginia of 300 persons.[23] He was also one of the "Ancient Adventurers" who petitioned "to have some men of qualitye sent Governor unto Virginia."[24] His interest in Virginia led to his appointment, December 13, 1620, as Physician General for the colony. With the position went an allotment of 500 acres of land and twenty

---

[21]Strachey: Travailes, p. 131.
[22]Stith: History of Virginia, p. 120.
[23]Records of the Virginia Company, v. 1, pp. 297, 303.
[24]Brown: Genesis of the U. S., v. 2, p. 830.

tenants, "to be placed thereupon at the companie's charge."[25]
About this time, also, he was appointed Councillor.

The Physician General sailed for Virginia in the *Margaret and John*. Somewhere in the West Indies a Spanish man of war appeared, and a stirring battle was fought. The little English sailing vessel outfought the Spaniard and made a safe getaway, but a shot from the enemy mortally wounded Dr. Bohun. An account of the battle was published in London under the title, "A True Relation of a Wonderfull Sea Fight between the great and well appointed Spanish Ships or men of Warre. And a small and not very well provided English Ship."[26] According to this story Dr. Bohun was caught in the arms of Captain Chester, who exclaimed, embracing him, "Oh, Dr. Bohun, what a disaster is this; the Noble Doctor no whit exanimated replyed, Fight it out, brave man, the cause is good, and the Lord receive my soule."

So perished one of the most colorful of early Virginia doctors, a man of talent, of an investigative nature, full of robust enthusiasm for the sea and for adventure. He had much in him to remind us of another seafaring physician, the buccaneer, Thomas Dover, who originated Dover's powders and was the terror of the Spanish Main. Bohun's widow petitioned the Company that, "as her husband in his lifetime was at great charge, as she supposes for the providing and transporting of servants into Virginia," she might

---

[25]Records of the Virginia Company, v. 1. p. 431.
[26]Brown: Genesis of the U. S., v. 2, p. 830.

be given some annual allowance. In the same petition she asked that her son, Edward Barnes, who was bound to serve the company for seven years, might be released. Both applications were rejected, the Company stating that it, and not Dr. Bohun, had borne the costs and charges and that Edward Barnes was the company's servant and could not be set free.[27]

The untimely death of Dr. Bohun did not discourage the Company in its effort to place the colony in the hands of well-trained medical men. The Company met immediately, and this is the record of what happened: "For so much as the physicians place to the Company was now become void by reason of the untimely death of Doctor Bohune slain in the fight with two Spanish Ships of War the 19th of March last; Doctor Gulstone did now take occasion to recommend unto the Company for the said place one Mr. Pottes, a Master of Arts and as he affirmed well practised in Chirurgerie and Phisique, and expert allso in distilling of waters and that he had many other ingenious devices so as he supposed his service would be of great use unto the Colony in Virginia, but prayed that whereas Doctor Bohune was tied by his contract to supply such of his tenants as should die after the first year at his own charge that Mr. Pottes might be relieved of that Covenant being too strict . . ." It was agreed that Dr. Pott should have the place on the same conditions as Dr. Bohun, with the addition of a "Chest of Phisique of 20 lb. and 10 lb. for books of phisique," which

27Encyclopedia of Virginia Biography, "Bohun."

Dr. Gulstone was to buy and charge to the Company; also free passage for Dr. Pott, his wife, a man and a maid, and for one or more chirurgeons, if they could be secured. These conditions were accepted by Dr. Pott on July 16, 1621.[28] In August the Council in England wrote Governor Yeardly in Virginia that "they had sent . . . Dr. John Potts for the phisition's place with two chirurgions and a chest of Physicke and Chirurgery."[29]

John Pott, although a man of education, was a contrast to his predecessor in many particulars. He seems to have had a taste for politics and affairs, and once in Virginia he stayed there.

During Dr. Pott's first year news reached England that the colonists, after making a treaty of peace with the Indians, had poisoned a great many of them, and that Dr. Pott was said to be "the chief actor in it." He was much blamed in England and lost the position he had held in the Council. The Earl of Warwick objected to his appointment, because he was "the poysoner of the salvages thear."[30]

A glimpse of the convivial disposition into which Pott appears to have retreated on occasion is given in a letter from George Sandys at Jamestown to a friend in London: "I have given from time to time the best councell I am able, at the first, he [Dr. Pott] kept companie too much with his inferiours, who hung upon him while his good liquor lasted.

[28]Records of the Virginia Company, v. 1, p. 517.
[29]Brown: First Republic, p. 454.
[30]Ibid., p. 639.

After, he consorted with Captaine Whitacres, a man of no good example, with whom he is gone into Kicotan, yet wheresoever he bee, he shall not bee without reach of my care, nor want for anything that I or my credit can procure him."[31]

In 1625 a petty quarrel brought the Doctor into court. The case illustrates the spirit of the times and the type of dispute that was often aired in the colonial courts of the Seventeenth Century. The *Minutes of the Council and General Court of Virginia* record that, "At a Court, May 9, 1625: Mrs. Elizabeth Hamer sworne and examined sayeth, yt [that] Mrs. Blany did miscary wth a Childe, but sayeth she doth not know whether Mrs. Blaynie did request a peece of hog flesh of Mr. Doctor Pott or nott, or that the wante of the peece of flesh was the occasione of her miscaryinge wth Childe, but sayeth yt Mrs. Blany did tell this Emamt [Examinent] yt she sent to Doctor Pott for A peece, and was denied.

"Mrs. Joane Peerce sworne and Examd sayeth yt Mrs. Blany cam to this examts house, requestinge her to send to Doctor Potts in her own name for A peece of hogs fflesh, Mrs. Blayny sayinge yt she had spoken to Doctor Pott for A peece, but was denyed it, and yt after[wards] Mrs. Blayny had miscaried, but ye tyme she knoweth not, nor whether yt were the occasione . . ."

Richard Townshend then testified that his master, Dr. Pott, had "apoynted his People to kill such hogs as tres-

---

[31]Neill: Virginia Carolorum, p. 79, footnote.

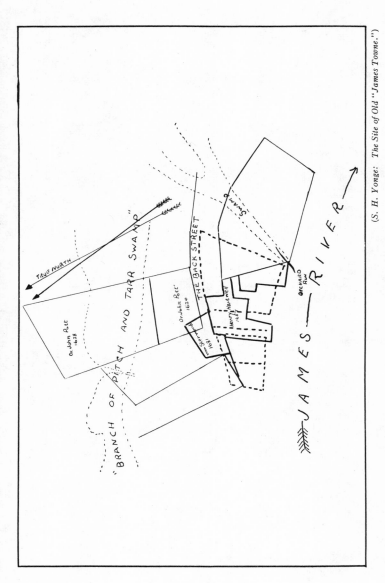

(S. H. Yonge: *The Site of Old "James Towne."*)

Map of portion of Jamestown, showing Dr. John Pott's holdings.

passed him in his Corne, and thervpon at severall tymes
they kild fower hogs wch were spent in his Mr [Master's]
house, but whose hogs they were, he knoweth nott . . ."
Several other witnesses testified as to the killing and eating
of the hogs at Dr. Pott's house.

The Court decided that "it is no slander yt Mrs. Blany
Chargeth Doctor Pott wth denying her a peece of fflesh,
wherevppon shee miscaried, because she hath taken her oath
that she thinketh in her Conscyenc that it was the occasion
of her miscaryinge, but it no way appereth, and it is bar-
barows to Imagine, that he had any conceipt she had A long-
ing to it but thought it was spent by his wiefe." "And for
ye hogs wose [whose] ever they were, the Courte conceveth
that there is no damage dew from Doctor Pott to the owner
of the hogs because the spoyle they did his Corne, was as
great as the valew of the hogs or greater. But his killinge
and eatinge of them without a legall order was irreguler and
Lyable to Censure, yet it appeares to be Publiqly done . . ."[32]

The following entry from the same court records shows
Dr. Pott acquiring land, and reference to the accompanying
map will show the property he eventually amassed in Jamestown proper. "Upon mocõn of Mr. Doctor Pott the Councell hath thought fitt and accordingly ordered that hee shall
have 200 acres of land between Kethe's Creeke and another
Creek adjoining."[33] Dr. Pott lived in that part of Jamestown called "Newtowne," on "Back Street," which was a

---

[32]Minutes of Council and General Court, pp. 58, 59.
[33]Ibid., p. 182.

continuation of "old Greate Road." Back Street was sixty
feet wide. His lot fronted twenty-five poles and contained
three acres. In 1628 he enlarged it by adding nine acres in
the rear. John Harvie lived across the way, and to the west
was Captain William Peirce, whose house was declared by
George Sandys, the poet, to be "the fairest in Virginia."
The poet had a room there, raised silk worms, and spent
his leisure translating Ovid. Pott, who is said to have understood Latin, Greek and Hebrew, was probably a congenial
neighbor.[34] In 1632 he was given 200 acres on Skiffe's
Creek, due for the "adventure" of four servants. He was
the first to locate land at the present site of Williamsburg.
His place there was called *Harrop* after the family estate
in Cheshire.

The names of several of Dr. Pott's servants have come
down to us. There were John Millwood, Thomas Gross,
Ruth, a maid servant, and Thomas Popkin. Thomas
Pritchard, aged 28, Thomas Lester, aged 33, and Roger
Stanley, aged 27, came over in the *Abigail* in 1620, and were
among "Dr. Pott's men" at the Main near Jamestown in
1624-25.[35] In 1625 another servant, Randall Holte, was
ordered by the Court to "serve and remain with Doctor Pott
his M'r until Christmas next-com twelve moneth. And then
Doctor Pott his m'r to deliver up his Indentures and make
him free, and to give him one suit of apparell from head to

---

[34]Tyler: Cradle of the Republic, p. 47.
[35]Virginia Magazine of History and Biography, v. 2, p. 185; v. 25, p. 125.

foote and three barrells of Corne."[36]   After the expiration
of his indentures Holt married Mary, daughter and heiress
of John Bayly, and acquired with her a large and valuable
tract of land on Hog Island.[37]

Richard Townshend was Dr. Pott's apprentice and afterwards became a distinguished member of the colony. Joseph
Fitch, the Doctor's apothecary, is listed as one of those massacred by the Indians in 1622.

Pott came to the colony with excellent professional recom-
mendations, and we have every reason to believe that he
lived up to them in spite of the maligning of his enemies.
His greatest enemy, Governor Harvey, wrote that he was
"skilled in the epidemical diseases" of the planters.   The
court records contain frequent references to his fees for
medical attendance.   In 1625 John Jefferson is ordered to
pay Dr. Pott "for Curynge of henry boothe's Eye."[38]   The
next year we find Stephen Tailor "being sicke and brought
home to Dr. Pott's his house."[39]   The hospitalization of
patients in the homes of physicians runs through the whole
century.

In 1626 Dr. Pott again appears in a lawsuit, this time with
Mr. Clayburne, Secretary of the colony.   The dispute concerned "certayne cowes" which the doctor claimed as his
own, "Appertaining to ye place of physition."   Pott was

---

[36]Minutes of Council and General Court, 1625, p. 98.
[37]Virginia Magazine of History and Biography, v. 25, p. 231.
[38]Minutes of Council and General Court, p. 84.
[39]Ibid., p. 155.

able to produce certificates to prove his point, and the court ordered that the cows should continue in his possession.[40]

In those days settlements were made along the James River, and transportation was largely by water. The woods were unsafe and the roads indifferent. In 1627 William Bennett was ordered to build Dr. Pott a boat.[41] He was probably a familiar figure on the James, his servants rowing him from one place of sickness to another.

Pott had been restored to his position in the Council, and when Governor West returned to England in 1629 he was elected temporary Governor. At a Court held in March 1628 there were present Dr. Pott, Captain Smythe, Captain Matthews, Mr. Secretary Ffarrar: "This daie the whole body of the council now remaining and resident in the colony did according to his Mats [Majesty's] letters patent assemble themselves and after full and serious consideration did elect and choose John Pott, Esqu. to be the present governor of and for this colony of Virginia."[42] For a year Virginia's first physician governor held the reins of authority. He twice convened the assembly, which consisted of the Governor, four councillors and forty-six burgesses, representing twenty-three plantations. Important regulations for the defence of the colony were adopted. Exports were becoming more and more important, and during 1629 no less than twenty-three ships visited Virginia waters. During Pott's

---

[40]Minutes of Council and General Court, pp. 161, 162.
[41]Ibid., p. 158.
[42]Ibid., p. 190.

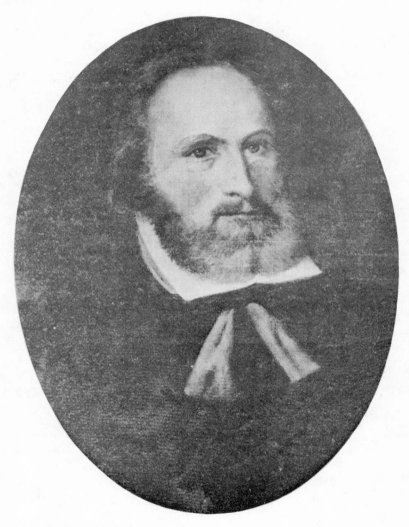

Lord Delaware, who complained of flux, cramps, ague and gout and whose
stay in Virginia was terminated by scurvy.

administration George Calvert, Lord Baltimore, landed at Jamestown, and would have stayed but for a chilly reception. Three years later he returned, but this time with a patent for Maryland.

In March 1630 Sir John Harvey arrived to become Governor. He at once took a dislike to Pott and soon had him arrested on three separate charges: "pardeninge willful murther; marking other men's Cattell for his owne and killing up their hoggs." The trial was conducted by a jury entirely under the coercion of the Governor, and it is not surprising that he was found guilty and his estates ordered confiscated. He was removed from the Council, and confined to his own plantation. Execution of the sentence was suspended, however, until the King's wish could be consulted.[43] Harvey rather inconsistently asked for clemency on the ground that Pott was the only physician in the colony capable of treating epidemic diseases. It is difficult to know the truth in this affair. Politics and jealousy and an anti-Pott faction in the colony probably loomed large behind the scenes. The King finally granted the Doctor's pardon.[44]

Pott returned to his practice but kept an eye on politics and on Governor Harvey. Harvey was one of Virginia's worst governors, and it was not long before trouble was brewing. Great discontent arose over his arbitrary conduct, especially in withholding petitions from the burgesses to the King. In 1634-35 secret meetings were organized by Dr.

[43]Minutes of Council and General Court, p. 479.
[44]Virginia Magazine of History and Biography, v. 8, pp. 33-35.

Pott's brother, Francis, and others. Dr. Pott was himself a leader in the popular discontent and assumed command of the musketeers while his brother circulated a petition against the Governor, calling for a redress of grievances.[45] The whole story is reminiscent of Bacon's Rebellion a generation later. Harvey quickly sensed the ringleader, arrested Dr. Pott, and put him in irons, but this time popular feeling was overwhelmingly with the Doctor. Governor Harvey was deposed and sent home to England, and John West was elected in his stead. Dr. Pott sailed for England on the same ship with Harvey, to present the colony's side of the case. But the King upheld his Governor and returned him to the colony. Pott remained in England, and continued to agitate against his old enemy. In 1639 he had the satisfaction of seeing Sir Francis Wyatt displace Harvey.

Dr. Pott died before 1642, for in that year the Court records mention 500 acres of land belonging to Francis Pott, "brother and heir" of John Pott.[46] He had figured largely in the life of the colony for more than twenty years.

Dr. Pott had a rather remarkable apprentice in Richard Townshend. Born about 1606, he came to Virginia at the early age of fourteen and in 1621 became an apprentice to Dr. Pott, to learn the art of an apothecary.[47] For six years he served his master faithfully, on one occasion witnessing for him in court. At the end of this time the young man

---

[45]Wertenbaker: Virginia under the Stuarts, pp. 74-84.
[46]Virginia Magazine of History and Biography, v. 1, p. 89.
[47]Ibid., v. 9, p. 173.

felt that Dr. Pott was neglecting his teaching and sought redress at a court held at "James Cittye," October 10, 1626: "Whereas at this Court there was petition made & preferred by Richard Townshend servant to Mr. Doctr Pott, against his Master, complaineing that he cannot bee Taught the art of an apothecarye, for the lerninge of wch art & misterye he was bond to ye said Doctr Pott by an Indenture bearing date the 20th day of ffebruary 1621, the Courte hath here-uppon ordered yt Mr. Doctor Pott doe henceforth from time to time endeavor to teach & instruct the said Richard Town-shend in ye art of an Apothecary by all convenient wayes & means he can or may, that soe hee may prove at ye end of his service a sufficient Apothecarye, wch if he ye said Mr. Doctr Pott shall neglect or refuse, the Court hath ordered yt he shall pay the said Richard Townshend for his service fro ye daye of ye date hereof unto the end and expiration thereof."[48]

Two years later (1628) we find Townshend a member of the House of Burgesses for "the Plantation between Archie's Hope and Martin's Hundred." From servant to Burgess in two years! Six years of study under the well-educated Dr. Pott set him above his fellows, among whom there was little of reading and writing. Pott, who was then Governor, evidently harbored no ill feeling for the affair in court two years before. Townshend advanced with phenomenal rapid-ity to the highest positions in the Colony. In 1630, when

---

[48]Minutes of Council and General Court, p. 117.

he was twenty-four years old, he is said to have moved with his wife, Frances, two white servants and three negro slaves to Keskyacke. In 1633 he was a Justice for York County. In 1636 he was appointed to the Council. In 1642 he was again a Burgess and a member of the Council, where his name appears until after 1645/6. Business called him to England frequently. He was there in 1635 and 1640, and in 1647 it is recorded that "Captain Richard Townsend, of Virginia, Esq., by God's Grace bound for England in the good ship *Honor,* of London," gave a power of attorney to his friend, Rowland Burnham. He owned considerable land, known as "Townsend Land," in York County. His son and heir, Francis,[49] came into possession of this in 1652, his father having died in the meantime. He lived a full life and died early, as did many of his contemporaries.[50]

The medical service of Captain William Norton would have been entirely forgotten but for Captain John Smith, who laments the death in the 1622 massacre of "Captaine Norton, a valiant, industrious Gentleman, adorned with many good qualities besides Physicke and Chirurgery, which for the publike good he freely imparted to all gratis, but most bountifully to the poore . . ."[51]—a rare trait in this age of blood and iron. Possibly it was the same Captain Norton who was associated with one of Virginia's earliest industries, the glass-works. His training in the sciences would have

---

[49]To his other son, Col. Robert Townshend, many Virginia families including Dades, Hooes, and Wallaces, trace their ancestry.
[50]Virginia Magazine of History and Biography, v. 9, p. 173.
[51]Smith: General History of Virginia, p. 586.

fitted him for the undertaking. The records of the Company show that "Intelligence was given that one Capt. Norton made an offer and would undertake to procure 6 strangers skilfull in makinge of Glasse and beads to goe over to Virginia to be employed in the saide work for the company for no other consideration than onely the half profits of their labors, and the said Norton would likewise go at his own charge and carry with him some servants and is contented to put himself upon the consideration of the company for what he shall have . . ." (June 1621).[52] In August the Council in London writes to Governor Yeardly in Virginia, recommending "Capt. Wm. Norton and his Italians, who go by this ship," and requesting the Governor to assist him in erecting his glass works. Though beads of glass are still found near Jamestown at the site of this early Virginia industry, the undertaking was of short duration. It yielded, like many another venture, to epidemic diseases and Indian tomahawks.

Among the medical men of this period was a "Master Cloybourne the Surgian." He arrived in October 1621 with Sir Francis Wyatt and Dr. Pott and was doubtless one of the two chirurgions the Physician General brought with him.[53] About this time, too, Mousnier de la Montagne, described as "medical student, marrying man," heads the list of a group of Walloons and French who offered "to go and inhabit in Virginia."

[52]Records of the Virginia Company, v. 1, p. 484.
[53]Smith: General History of Virginia, p. 564.

Robert Pawlett was one of those parson physicians of whom Virginia had not a few. He combined the threefold capacities of preacher, physician and surgeon, and he sailed for Virginia in September 1619 under an agreement with the Company. In 1621 he was elected to the Council but declined to serve because "the adventurers of Martin's Hundred felt that their business required his presence continually."[54] He was preacher at Berkeley Hundred in 1621 and is supposed to have died before 1623.

Another surgeon whose life was of short tenure in the colony was William Rowsley, who arrived early in 1623 with his wife and ten men, after receiving a patent in 1622. In a short period all of them were dead.[55]

Of another doctor nothing remains but an inscription in stone, found in the vicinity of a former Indian village on Potomac Creek, in what is now Stafford County.[56] On the tombstone in rough letters one and three-quarters inches long had been inscribed:

HERE LIES INTERED
THE BODY OF EDMOND
HELDER PRECTIONER IN
PHYSICK AND CHIRURGE
RY. BORN IN BEDFORDE
SHIRE   OBIIT MARCH 11
1618. S. ATATIS SUA 76

54Neill: Virginia Vetusta, p. 174.
55Ibid., p. 121. Records of the Virginia Company, v. 2, p. 91.
56Harper's Magazine, Jan. 1886.

This is the earliest tombstone of a physician dying in this
country and, with a possible single exception, the earliest
English tombstone of any sort.

In the latter years of the London Company's control of
Virginia the names of three chirurgeons appear among the
"divers ancient Planters, Mrs of Shipps, Marriners, and

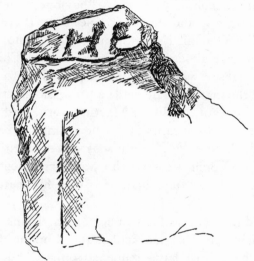

Fragment of Helder's Tombstone.—*Harper's Magazine.*

sundry other persons that had lived long in Virginia and
have been many tymes there."[57]   They were signers of a
rebuttal to Captain Butler's slanderous account of the colony
in 1622.   The first was William Green, a chirurgeon, who
had lived seventeen months in Virginia.   Two years later he

[57]Neill: Virginia Company of London, pp. 394-403.

was in court collecting a bill of "Phisick & surgery" for services to John Stephens, "himself and his servants at sea."[58] He had earlier been described as "Chirurgion in the *Temperance*." Evidently ship surgeons practised on land and often took up their abode for months in the colony, where they owned property. The second signer was Henry Hitch, "Chirurgeon of ye *James*," "havinge been 2 severall times in Virginia and lived at one time there about 5 monneths." The third was Samuel Mole, who had lived "3 years or ther aboutes in Virginia beinge a Chirurgion."

Edward Gibson was apparently a physician, for in 1622, just before the massacre, he made a professional trip to Falling Creek: "Capt. Nicholas Martin sworne and examined saith that Ed: Gibson cam upp to the fallinge Creek, administered Phisick to ev'y of the p'sons specified, then went & did that Cure uppon Fossett who was farre spent with the droppsie . . . and not one of these his patients misc[arried]."[59]

We have the names of a number of physicians who practised medicine in Virginia under the London Company. Many of them must have remained only a short time or fallen a prey to the high mortality, for the colony was often in dire straits for medical aid. In 1610 a "Table of such as are required to this Plantation" is appended to "A True and Sincere Declaration of the Purpose and Ends of the Plantation begun in Virginia . . . Set forth by the authority

---

[58]Minutes of Council and General Court, p. 65.
[59]Ibid., in Virginia Magazine of History and Biography, v. 19, p. 144.

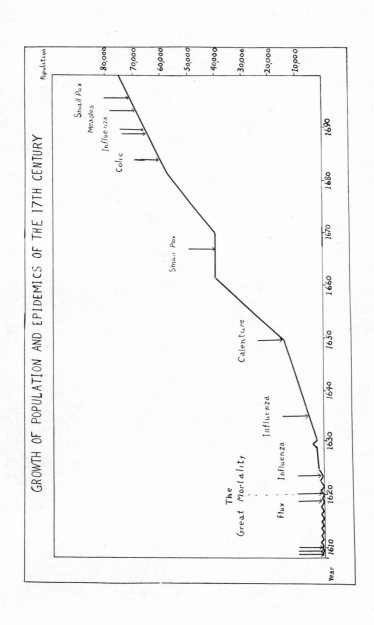

GROWTH OF POPULATION AND EPIDEMICS OF THE 17TH CENTURY

of the Governor and Councellors established for that Plantation." The Table includes: "Foure honest and learned Ministers, 2 Surgeons, 2 Druggists," together with various other occupations.[60] Sir Thomas Dale wrote to the Virginia Company, May 25, 1611: "Our wante likewise of able chirurgions is not a little, be pleased to advise the committee for us in this pointe."[61] At another time the Court "receaved letters from Virginia importinge the wellfare of the Plantation although they have been much distemperd by reason of an intemporate heate . . . requestinge that the Company would send them some Phisitians and Apothycaries of which they stand much need off . . ."[62]

The regime of the London Company ended in 1624. It had shown a rather high conception of the type of physician that should be sent to the colony. Russell, Bohun, Pott and Pawlett were all men of education. Throughout the remaining years of the century Virginia had many physicians and surgeons, most of them home grown, self educated, or products of a local apprenticeship. There were probably none comparable in training and education to the men sent over by the London Company before 1624. In the days of her greatest mortality, when epidemic diseases were decimating the ranks of the new adventurers, Virginia had the advantage of medical talent which probably represented a fair cross-section of contemporary British medicine.

---

[60]Brown: Genesis of the U. S., v. 1, p. 353.
[61]Ibid., p. 493.
[62]Records of the Virginia Company, v. 1, p. 310.

CHAPTER II

EPIDEMIC DISEASES

I

Population and Mortality

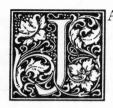AMESTOWN was settled in 1607 with 105 colonists. By the end of the century, after many vicissitudes, the population had grown to approximately 75,000. That this was a disappointing increase is shown in the report of Edward Randolph to the Board of Trade.[1] More than 100,000 Englishmen had immigrated to Virginia before 1700.[2] There must have been a considerable increment to the population through births, a multiparous motherhood balancing a high infant mortality. Yet, after a hundred years of colonization, in spite of a normal addition to population through births, there were living in Virginia 25,000 fewer persons than had immigrated.

There was a steady flow of immigrants from England throughout the Seventeenth Century. The average yearly increase from this source was 1,750. Of this number 1,500 were indentured servants, who after the usual period of five years became freedmen and soon dominated the colony

---

[1]British Public Record Office CO5-1362, pp. 369-373, Colonial Entry Book, cited by Wertenbaker, Planters of Colonial Virginia, p. 177.
[2]Wertenbaker: Planters of Colonial Virginia, pp. 36-41.

numerically.[3] The Virginia planter of the Seventeenth Century unlike his successor of the Eighteenth was of the yeo-
man class, owning and cultivating small plantations. Before
1660 conditions were favorable to the development of the
small planter. Later, two factors became more and more
destructive of his interests—the navigation laws disastrously
reduced the price of tobacco, and negro slavery became more
firmly established. The result was a great migration of
small planters out of Virginia into North Carolina, Maryland and Pennsylvania. This exodus was one reason for the
slow growth of Seventeenth Century Virginia. The chief
reason was the high mortality which prevailed throughout
the Century.

In the early years at Jamestown, before 1618, 1,100 out
of 1,700 immigrants perished. Sixty died the first summer,
twenty the next, seventeen the next. Then came the fatal
year, 1610, when 338 died, reducing the colony to sixty souls.
Six hundred and sixty-five died between 1610 and 1618.
This was said to be a healthy period! Six hundred were
left in Virginia.[4]

After 1618 the number of immigrants increased, averag-
ing more than a thousand a year. But in February 1625
only 1,095 remained out of 7,549.[5] Not one out of six had

[3]Wertenbaker: Planters of Colonial Virginia, pp. 36-41.
[4]Brown: First Republic, p. 285.
[5]Ibid. 1700 came to Virginia before 1618 (p. 285)
        840 came in 1618-19   (p. 329)
       4749 came between 1619-1624   (p. 612)
        260 came in 1624-25   (p. 612)

       7549 total of immigrants before 1625

survived. There is no record of any such decimating mortality after this, though the slow growth of population up to
1649 would indicate that the hazards of life in Virginia were
still extreme.   In 1635 there were only 4,914 inhabitants,[6]
in 1649 the number rose to 15,000,[7] and in 1662 it was
40,000.[8] In 1671 Governor Berkeley reported improved
health conditions—the newcomers now rarely failed to sur-
vive the "seasoning period," whereas formerly about twenty
percent had succumbed during their first months in the new
country.[9]   Nevertheless, the population was practically
stationary between 1660-70, due chiefly, perhaps, to economic and social causes.   By 1681 it had risen to 56,000,
and by the end of the century it was variously estimated as
between 60,000 and 75,000.

II

The Voyage from England

The immigrant to Virginia encountered hazards to his
health long before he reached the shores of the colony.
Deaths on shipboard were frequent, due often to improper
diet, sometimes to disease, again to outbreaks of epidemic
disorders. Gabriel Archer wrote in 1609 that "out of two
ships was thrown overboard 32 persons," and one vessel lost
130 out of 185 of her passengers on her voyage to Vir-

[6]Calendar British State Papers, v. 1574-1660, p. 201.
[7]U. S. Census, 1910, v. 3, p. 913n.
[8]British Museum, Egerton MSS. 2395, f356b (Wertenbaker: Planters
of Colonial Virginia.)
[9]Hening: Statutes at Large, v. 2, p. 515.

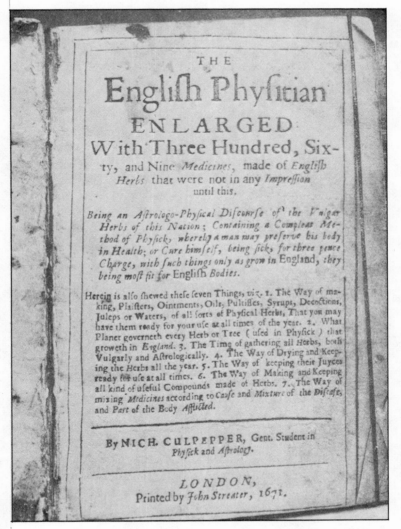

THE

English Phyſitian

ENLARGED

With Three Hundred, Six-
ty, and Nine *Medicines*, made of *Engliſh*
Herbs that were not in any *Impreſſion*
until this.

Being an *Aſtrologo-Phyſical Diſcourſe* of the *Vulgar*
Herbs of this *Nation*; Containing a *Compleat Me-*
thod of Phyſick, whereby a man may preſerve his body
in Health; or Cure himſelf, being ſick, for three pence
Charge, with ſuch things only as grow in England, they
being moſt fit for Engliſh *Bodies*.

Herein is alſo ſhewed theſe ſeven Things, viz. 1. The Way of making, Plaiſters, Ointments, Oils, Pultiſſes, Syrups, Decoctions,
Juleps or Waters, of all ſorts of Phyſical Herbs, That you may
have them ready for your uſe at all times of the year. 2. What
Planet governeth every Herb or Tree (uſed in Phyſick) that
groweth in *England*. 3. The Time of gathering all Herbs, both
Vulgarly and Aſtrologically. 4. The Way of Drying and Keeping the Herbs all the year. 5. The Way of keeping their Juyces
ready for uſe at all times. 6. The Way of Making and Keeping
all kind of uſeful Compounds made of Herbs. 7. The Way of
mixing *Medicines* according to *Cauſe* and *Mixture* of the *Diſeaſes*,
and Part of the Body *Afflicted*.

By NICH. CULPEPPER, Gent. Student in
Phyſick and Aſtrology.

LONDON,
Printed by *John Streater*, 1671.

Title page of Culpeper's *English Physician*, a book often found in
Seventeenth Century Virginia libraries.

ginia.[10] As late as 1636 Governor West reported to the authorities in England, "I find with all that muche imputation indeservedly lyeth upon the Countrye, by the Merchants crime whoe soe pester their shipps with passengers, that through throng and noysomeness they bring noe lesse than infection among us which is soe easily to be distinguished from any cause in the malignitie of the clymate, that where the most pestered shipps vent their passengers they carry with them almost a general mortallitye."[11]

In a letter to the President and Council of the Company in 1611 Sir Thomas Dale advises the passage to Virginia by way of Dominico, in order to bring about "restitution of our sick people into health by the helpes of Fresh ayre, diet and the baths. For true it is we being understripped of Tonnage, and pestered by that means, that our goods filled up the Orlage having no room for our men to be accommodated, but crowded together their own aires and the uncleanliness of the ship, dogs, etc., gave some infexion amongst us & was the cause of the loss of well more a dozen men."[12] But that very habit of visiting the Antilles exposed the passengers and sailors to tropical diseases that later broke out on shipboard, infected their water buckets with mosquito larvae, and so laid the stage for carrying disease into the colony. When the ships ran a southerly course, "many of our men fell sick of the calenture."

---

[10]Brown: Genesis of the U. S., p. 329.
[11]Neill: Virginia Carolorum, p. 130.
[12]Ibid., p. 489.

Constant complaints of these pestered ships were made to the authorities at home. In 1624 the governor and council in Virginia blamed the condition of the ships for the death of new comers,[13] and Governor Wyatt and thirty others the same year replied to questions asked by commissioners from England that "a care must be had that the ships come not over pestered and that they may be well used at sea with that plenty and goodness of dyet as is promised in England but seldom performed; a proportion of mault they should also bring over to make themselves beer, that the sudden drinking of water cause not too great alteration in their bodyes."[14]

In 1623 the governor and council wrote the Earl of Southampton of the great loss of men through infection, chiefly brought in by the ships, and requested that strict orders might be given for proper provisioning. They also complained that "Dupper's beer" had been the death of a great number.[15] Dupper was an English brewer. About this same time George Sandys remarked that "the country will be pleased to hear that revenge has been taken of Dupper for his stinking beer, which has been the death of 200 persons."[16] According to another contemporary account: "The mortality which is imputed to the country alone is chiefly caused by the pestered ships which reach Virginia victualled with musty bread and stinking beer."[17] As late as

---

[13]Brown: First Republic, p. 569.
[14]Ibid., p. 578.
[15]Calendar British State Papers, v. 1574-1660, p. 41.
[16]Ibid., p. 43.
[17]Ibid., p. 56.

1680 Lord Culpeper, arriving in Virginia, writes of "a most tedious passage of eleven weeks and two days, full of death, scurvy and calentures."[18]

The slow sailing vessels of those days, requiring two or three months to cross the Atlantic and often taking the southern route by the Barbadoes, were potent means of introducing disease and epidemics into Virginia. They embarked from epidemic centres in England, were overcrowded, had poor sanitary arrangements, carried open fire buckets which might harbor mosquito larvae, and were inadequately provisioned, especially in the matter of citrous fruits to prevent scurvy.[19]

III

"Seasoning"

The immigrant who survived his passage from England had to face what was known in Virginia as the "seasoning." This usually came in the summer and was attributed to many causes. According to DeVries, during "June, July and August . . . people that have lately arrived from England die . . . like cats and dogs, whence they call it the sickly season."[20] Immigrants soon learned that in order to avoid the "summer sickness," as the seasoning was sometimes called, it was best to reach Virginia in the fall and winter. In this way they escaped the hot summer sun of the tropics

---

[18]Virginia Magazine of History and Biography, v. 25, p. 139.
[19]Citrous fruit for scurvy was a prophylactic receipt known to Sir Richard Hawkins in 1593 and to Commodore James Lancaster in 1600.
[20]Wertenbaker: Virginia under the Stuarts, p. 12.

en route and had time to become "hardened" in Virginia before the advent of the sickly season of the next summer.[21] Undoubtedly the hot suns of the Virginia summer, especially in the tobacco fields, went very hard with the indentured servant, unaccustomed to such heat, undernourished after a long sea voyage, and often the host of an infectious disease bred in his new environment.

Purchas lists as causes of the calamitous summers: lack of houses and victuals, "brackish, slimey water at James Fort, . . . Sending ill People that consumed the rest with idlenesse; . . . Sicknesse caused by the grosse and vaporous Aire and soyle about James Towne, and drinking water."[22] Strachey, who travelled through Virginia in 1610 and was well informed on colonial matters, gives his opinion that "the temperature of this country doth well agree with the English constitutions, being sometymes seasoned in the same, which hath appeared unto us by this, that albeyt, by many occasions, ill lodging at the first (the poorer on the bare ground, and the best in such miserable cotages at the best, as through which the piercing heat of the sun, which there (it is true) is the first cause, creating such sommer fevers amongst them, found never resistaunce) hard fare, and their owne judgements and saffeties instructing them to worke hard in the faint tyme of sommer (the better to be accomodated and fitted for the wynter,) they have fallen sick, yet have they recovered agayne, by very small meanes,

---

21Neill: Virginia Company of London, p. 276.
22Purchas: Pilgrimage, p. 833.

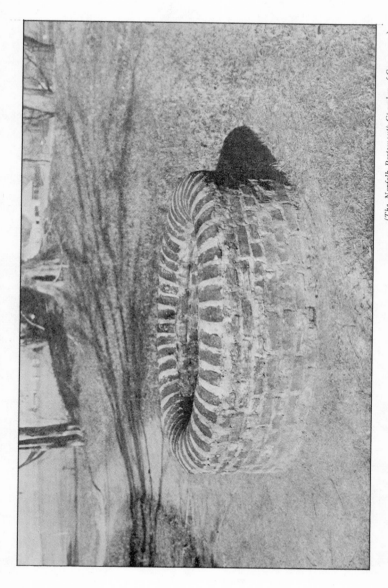

The well at Jamestown as it appears today. Sickness and death lurked here in the Seventeenth Century.

without helpe of fresh diet, or comfort of wholesome physique, there being at the first but few physique helpes, or
skilfull surgeons, who knew how to apply the right medicine
in a new country, or to search the quality and constitution
of the patient, and his distemper, or that knew how to councell, when to lett blood, or not, or in necessity to use a launce
in that office at all."[23]

The fatal summers of 1607 and 1608 gave to the seasoning a grave significance which is voiced in all the writings of
the earlier observers. Toward the end of the century it was
viewed with less apprehension. In 1671 Governor Berkeley
replied to the inquiries of the Lords Commissioners about
the death rate in the colony, "All new plantations are, for
an age or two, unhealthy, 'till they are thoroughly cleared
of wood; but unless we had a particular register office for
the denoting of all that died, I cannot give a particular answer to this query, only this I can say, that there is not often
unseasoned hands (as we term them) that die now, whereas
heretofore, not one of five escaped the first year."[24]

A letter from William Fitzhugh to Dr. Ralph Smith in
1687 shows the loose way in which the term "seasoning" was
used at that time: "I take this last opportunity by way of
London to acquaint you that now praised be God we are all
in good health, my Sister has had her Seasoning, if it may be
so called, two or three fits of feaver & ague which almost a
week since has left, but yet she is a little undisposed to

---

[23]Strachey: Travailes, p. 30.
[24]Hening: Statutes at Large, v. 2, p. 515.

write."[25]   As late as 1723 we find George Hume, a recent
arrival in Virginia, writing to a relative in Scotland: "We
had no sooner landed in this Country, but I was taken immediately wth all ye most common distempers yt attend it,
but ye most violent of all was a severe flux of wch my uncle
died, being the governor's factor at a place called Ger-
mawna. . . . All that comes to this country have ordinarly
sickness at first wch they call a seasoning of wch I shall as-
sure you I had a most severe one when I went to town. . ."[26]

Beverley explains the "fluxes, fevers and the bellyache"
that greeted newcomers by the fact that they "greedily surfeit with their delicious fruits, and are guilty of great intemperance therein, through the exceeding plenty thereof,
and liberty given by the inhabitants; by which means they
fall sick, and then unjustly complain of the unhealthiness of
the country. . . . Exercise and a bright sun made them hot,
and then they imprudently fell to drinking cold water, or
perhaps new cider, which, in its season they found in every
planter's house; or else they greedily devour the green fruit,
and unripe trash they met with, and so fell into fluxes, fevers,
and the bellyache; . . . This is the true state of the case,
as to the complaints of its being sickly; for, by the most
impartial observation I can make, if people will be persuaded
to be temperate, and take due care of themselves, I believe
it is as healthy a country as any under heaven; but the extra-

25Virginia Magazine of History and Biography, v. 2, p. 142.
26William and Mary Quarterly, v. 6, p. 254.

ordinary pleasantness of the weather, and plenty of the fruit, lead people into many temptations."[27]

Evidently the seasoning was much more serious in the first decades of the life of the colony. Its chief causes were "pestered" ships where undernourishment and disease worked havoc before the immigrant arrived; poor food; crowded, unsanitary living conditions at the port of entry, where lurking epidemic diseases got periodic fresh starts; and, finally, hard work in the sun for raw hands.

IV

War, Famine and Pestilence

The disappointing growth of population in Seventeenth Century Virginia has been dealt with by historians and economists but has never been analyzed from a medical point of view. However important the economic and social factors, it can hardly be denied that the main set-backs to Virginia's growth in man power in the Seventeenth Century were untimely deaths which had their origin in war, famine and pestilence. It is difficult to estimate precisely and separately the death rate from these three factors. It is probably safe to say that prior to 1612 food deficiency was the major cause of the high mortality. After that, disease far outranked all other factors, although Indian warfare also took a steady and decisive toll of human life.

Thousands of colonists undoubtedly lost their lives dur-

[27]Beverley: History of Virginia, ch. 19.

ing this century in Indian warfare and from accidents.
Eight were killed the first year,[28] sixty-four were massacred
in 1609,[29] 347 lost their lives in the great massacre of
1622.[30] Captain Henry Spelman and twenty-six of his men
perished in 1624, and from three to five hundred were
massacred in 1644.[31] Numbers fell at the unfortunate de-
feat at Bloody Run, and sixty of Mason and Brent's men
were killed in 1675.[32] Thirty-six deaths are recorded the
next year from Indian raids on the upper Potomac.[33] There
was great loss of life all along the frontier during the period
of Bacon's Rebellion, and Governor Berkeley hanged
twenty-three of Bacon's followers after the death of their
leader. We can thus account for well over a thousand
deaths during little more than half the century. There
must have been innumerable others in the daily frontier
clash between the resentful redskins and the whites who
were ever trespassing on their domain.

The loss of life from food deficiency was due not only to
lack of food but to dietary diseases which were sequellae of
poorly balanced rations. The poor and insufficient food on
shipboard has already been mentioned. George Percy in
his list of the causes of death in 1607 remarked, "For the
most part they died of meere famine. . . . Our food was but

---

[28]Smith: General History of Virginia, pp. 95-6.
[29]Stanard: Story of Virginia's First Century, pp. 87-90.
[30]Colonial Records of Virginia, State Senate Document.
[31]Stanard: Story of Virginia's First Century, pp. 176, 209.
[32]Ibid., pp. 231, 260.
[33]Ibid., p. 260.

a small can of Barlie sod in water to five men a day."[34]
Stith writes of the winter of 1609-10, "In short, so extreme
was the Famine and Distress of this time, that it was, for
many Years after, distinguished and remembered, by the
Name of the Starving Time. And by these means, of near
five hundred Persons, left by Captain Smith at his Depar-
ture, within six Months, there remained not above sixty,
Men, Women, and Children; and these most poor and miserable Creatures, preserved, for the most part, by Roots,
Herbs, Acorns, Walnuts, Berries, and now and then a little
Fish. Neither was it possible for them, to have held out
ten days longer, without being utterly extinct and famished
with Hunger."[35]

Later in the century the author of *Leah and Rachel* declares, "I believe it was only want of such diet as best agreed
with our English natures . . . were the cause of so much
sicknesses, as were formerly frequent, which we have now
amended."[36] In 1623 the Company complained by letter
that they were much grieved by the mortality which had
persisted since the massacre, and expressed their belief that
it "proceeded in great part through distempers and disorders in dyet and lodginge."[37]

In 1613 Gondomar wrote to Philip of Spain, "There are
about three hundred men there more or less; and the ma-

---

[34]Percy: Discourse. Reprinted in Brown: Genesis of the U. S., v. 1,
p. 168.
[35]Stith: History of Virginia, p. 117.
[36]Force: Tracts, v. 3, "Leah & Rachel," p. 10.
[37]Neill: Virginia Company of London, p. 392.

jority sick and badly treated, because they have nothing to
eat but bread of maize with fish; nor do they drink anything but water—all of which is contrary to the nature of
the English—on which account they all wish to return and
would have done so if they had been at liberty."[38]

The answer of the General Assembly in 1623/4 to Alder-
man Johnson's praise of Sir Thomas Smith's government of
the colony may have been a bit prejudiced: "In those twelve
years of Sir Thomas Smith's government the Colony for
the most part remained in great want and misery. . . .
That the allowance for a man in those times, was only eight
ounces of meal and half a pint of pease a day, both the one
and the other being moldy, rotten, full of cobwebbs and
maggots, loathsome to man. . . . That others were forced,
by famine, to filch for their bellies. . . . That if a man,
through sickness had not been able to work, he had no allowance at all, and so consequently perished. That their
scarcity was sometimes so lamentable that they were constrained to eat dogs, cats, rats, snakes, toadstools, horse-
hides, and what not. That one man, out of the misery he
endured, killed his wife, and powdered her up to eat; for
which he was burnt: That many others fed on the corpses
of dead men. . . ."[39]

On the other hand "A True Declaration of the estate of
the Colonie in Virginia," published by order of the Council
of Virginia in 1610, says that the stories of famine were

---

[38]Brown: Genesis of the U. S., p. 660.
[39]Journals House of Burgesses, v. 1619-1658/9, pp. 21, 22.

untrue and originated with a group of the colonists who banded themselves together as pirates and later returned to England, having agreed among themselves to tell the same story of famine and to protest that "this their comming awaie, proceeded from desperate necessitie: These are they, that roared out the tragicall historie of the man eating of his dead wife in Virginia. . . ."[40]

Sir Thomas Gates explained this story as follows: "There was one of the companie who mortally hated his wife, and therefore secretly killed her . . . and . . . to excuse himselfe he said that his wife died, that he hid her to satisfie his hunger, and that he fed daily upon her.   Upon this, his house was againe searched, where they found a good quantitie of meale, oatemeale, beanes and pease.   Hee thereupon was arraigned, confessed the murder, and was burned for his horrible villany."[41]

Some famine there undoubtedly was in the early years of the colony, and a search for its causes does not take one far afield.   The ships were poorly provisioned when they sailed, and the voyage was a long one.   On landing, the new settlers found very little to support life, and were slow in learning to clear the land and to plant sufficient food for their needs.   Indeed, the planters felt the pinch of hunger before the ships which brought them had sailed on the return voyage, and many of them bartered with sailors for biscuits in return for sassafras and other Virginia products.

---

[40]Force: Tracts, v. 3, "A True Declaration etc.," p. 16.
[41]Ibid.

The planters were forbidden to cultivate land on their own
initiative until Governor Dale's time. As late as 1610 the
whole corn crop amounted to but seven acres, and it is
stated that Lord Delaware's men had devoured the whole
crop three days after they landed, so famished were they
for fresh green vegetables and so improvident of the future.
It is probable that famine and starvation were not real
problems in the colony after these early years. During the
summer of 1611 Henricopolis was laid out and Bermuda
Hundred palisaded, affording protection for new plantations projected on a wide scale. With the laying out of new
plantations and with an ever widening frontier the food
problem ceased to be acute and is not mentioned again until
1622, when the Indian massacre made frontier life so
hazardous that many planters withdrew into the ancient
fortified centers.

These early years of hardship were favorable to the development of food deficiency diseases, and contemporary
descriptions which record them as having assumed epidemic
proportions both on shipboard and among the early settlers
have considerable medical interest. Such diseases are naturally latent, often requiring months of improper rationing
before making their appearance. They are also subtle and,
masquerading as swellings, fail entirely to suggest to the
victims their real etiology. The two such diseases that
affected the colony were beriberi and scurvy.

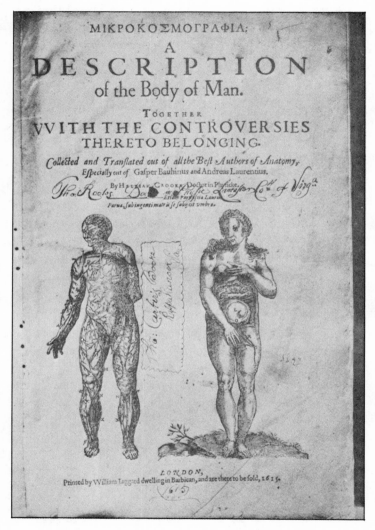

Title page of the copy of Crooke's *Body of Man* owned in the
Seventeenth Century by Dr. Thomas Rootes, and bearing his
signature: "Tho: Rootes. Doctor in Physic, Lancaster,
Coll of Virga."

V

Beriberi[42]

Percy, cataloguing the mortality at Jamestown in 1607, heads the list of "cruell diseases" with "Swellings." His reference was probably to beriberi, sometimes called epidemic dropsy, the twin sister of those other accompaniments of insufficient and unbalanced rations: scurvy and starvation. Certain Indian tribes doubtless had beriberi. The early settlers were warned to avoid localities in which the natives showed large bellies and strange swellings.[43] Though beriberi as a name was not coined until Bonitus used it in 1758, Strabo described it among the armies of Rome in 24 B. C., and early descriptions of it are found in Chinese and Japanese literature. Only recently, unbalanced rations aboard the German raider, *Kronprinz Wilhelm,* led to beriberi, and accomplished what the combined fleets of the Allies had failed to do.

Beriberi, as is now well known, is a dietary deficiency disease. Stith says that the people of Jamestown were "reduced to a common kettle which contained the allowance of half a pint of wheat and as much barley boiled with water for a man a day. This having funked for six and twenty weeks in the ship's hold contained nothing substantial, being only Bran with as many worms as grains." In this common

---

[42]A Singalese term meaning "I cannot," used in the sense of "I am too ill to do anything," is quite descriptive of the colony to which Smith returned.

[43]Neill: Virginia Company of London, p. 12.

pot lie all the etiological factors of beriberi. The anti-neuritic vitamine, so-called B, was undoubtedly lacking in the mouldy, rat-eaten barley which was the basis of the pot, and long boiling may have destroyed what little there was to begin with. The preventative of the disease—eggs, vegetables and fruits—the colonists did not have. Stith was probably right, therefore, in his conclusion that the early mortality was due to food and hardships rather than to infectious disease: "This unwholesome Food, together with their continued toil and Labour in the Extremity of Heat, carried off fifty of the Company by September."

Beriberi is often characterized by swelling—the so-called dropsical form. Fluid under the skin and in the body cavities produces a general anasarca and the victim presents a typical swelling. There are also the dry forms, and these might well be portrayed in the "anatomies" which were described in the streets of Jamestown during this calamitous year, 1607. Castellani calls attention to the fact that acute pernicious types of beriberi occur, "when the person, without previous illness, suddenly dies." Some of the first planters are said to have died suddenly and without obvious cause, and this is doubtless the explanation.

VI

Scurvy

Whereas beriberi was unknown to the medical profession in the Seventeenth Century, scurvy had been recognized from the earliest times as a disease prone to affect mariners.

Vasco da Gama lost 100 of his 156 men as a result of scurvy, before he reached the Cape of Good Hope, and though its cure was known as early as the Sixteenth Century there were 30,000 cases in our own Civil War. It is not surprising, therefore, to find the colonists developing it both on the long voyage to America and after their arrival in Virginia. In 1610 Lord Delaware complained of "the disease called scurvy; which though in others it be a sicknesse of slothfulnesse, yet was in me an effect of weaknesse, which never left me, till I was upon the point to leave the world." On advice of his physician, Dr. Bohun, he sought a cure in the West Indies, where "I found help for my health and my sicknesse assuaged, by means of fresh dyet and especially of Oranges and Lemonds, an undoubted remedy and medicine for that disease."[44] During the same winter an Indian died of scurvy at Jamestown.[45]

On account of the number of immigrants who suffered from scurvy at sea Dr. John Woodall, the medical adviser to Sir Thomas Smith, gave it his special attention. He was a "Master in Chirurgerie," and in 1636 published *The Surgeon's Mate,* the earliest book in which lemon juice was prescribed for scurvy.

Captain Ralph Hamor after five years' residence in the colony declared that few idlers escaped "the scurvy disease, with which few or none, once infected, have recovered."[46]

[44]Brown: Genesis of the U. S., v. 1, pp. 479, 480.
[45]Brown: First Republic, p. 137.
[46]Hamor: A True Discourse of the Present State of Virginia, p. 19.

Scurvy is a disease characterized by mental apathy and lassitude and painful joints. It is interesting that a disease which would so naturally have occasioned the appearance of idleness should have had idleness assigned to it as its cause.

There was undoubtedly a sprinkling of scurvy in the colony all through the century. Chirurgeon John Peteet, of York County, was a member of a coroner's jury, October 24, 1659, which found after an inquest that "the corps was very much diseased" and that "this disease being ye scourvey was ye cause of his death."[47] In 1675 a Surry County jury reported that a runaway maid servant died "by reason of a distemper called the Scurvy."[48]

A strange disease of the skin is described by Smith as affecting his whole party on one of their journeys inland. The skin of their entire bodies peeled off, as if they had been flayed from head to foot. This must have been a form of dermatitis exfoliativa, of either metabolic or infectious origin.

VII

Malaria

A theory advocated by W. H. S. Jones, that the decline and fall of Greek civilization was due to malaria, has had considerable vogue. This assertion has encountered vigorous protest and denial of late from Greek physicians. Vir-

---

[47]York County Records, v. 3, p. 173.
[48]Surry County Records, v. 2, p. 95.

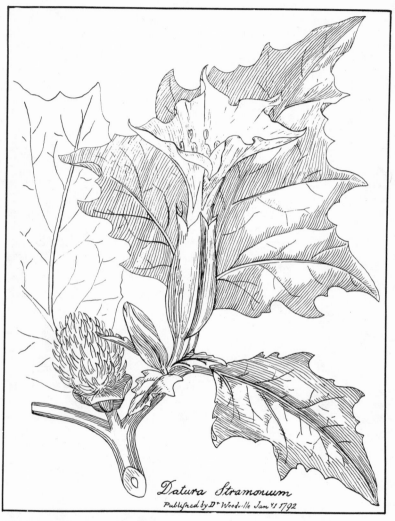

Datura Stramonium
Published by Dr Woodville Jany 1.st 1792

Jimson or Jamestown Weed, which grew on the open lots about the first colony, and was early recognized as medicinally potent.

ginia's historians have for the most part attributed the early severe mortality in the colony to the same disease. There are repeated references to the prevalence and fatality of malaria. Thus, "Swarms of mosquitoes arose from the stagnant pools of water to attack the immigrants with a sting more deadly than that of the Indian arrow or Spanish musket ball. Scarcely three months had elapsed from the first landing when sickness and death made their appearance. The settlers, ignorant of the use of Peruvian bark and other remedies, were powerless to resist the progress of the epidemic. . . . So deadly was the epidemic that when Captain Newport brought relief in January, 1608, he found but thirty-eight of the colonists alive."[49] Again, "Malaria was rampant and quinine unknown."[50] The fearful mortality of the first years is said by another historian to have been fought without avail "because the only specific, quinine, was yet unknown."[51] Such sweeping statements about malaria in Virginia do not appear to be borne out by the facts.

The contemporary sources of Seventeenth Century Virginia history contain few references to diseases which might be called malaria. Percy, whose full account of the first mortality at Jamestown is frequently quoted, refers to "swellings, flixes and burning fevers" but not to the ague. Had the ague (malaria) with its racking chills been present, contemporary writers who were fond of describing diseases

---

[49]Wertenbaker: Virginia under the Stuarts, p. 11.
[50]Stanard: Story of Virginia's First Century, p. 43.
[51]Brown: First Republic, p. 380.

by their outstanding symptoms would hardly have failed to mention it. We have been able to find in the original sources for this century only five or six actual references to the ague.

Lord Delaware writes in 1610: "presently after my arrival in Jamestowne, I was welcomed by a hot and violent ague, which held mee a time, till by the advice of my Physition, Doctor Lawrence Bohun, (by blood letting), I was recovered. . . ."[52] Strachey declared in 1610 that there were "many diseases and sicknesses which have happened to our people, who are indeede strangely afflicted with Fluxes and Agues; and every particular season . . . hath his particular infirmities too."[53] In the absence of the therapeutic test by quinine, which did not come into the colony before the middle of the century, and of modern blood examinations, which were not in practise until 1890, the term "ague" is vague and might cover a multitude of febrile diseases.[54] In 1687 William Fitzhugh wrote that his sister had "2 or 3 fitts of a fever and ague." A deposition in the Henrico County records for 1688 discloses that one John Womeck, when his wife "had a violent Feaver and Ague on her" did

---

[52]Brown: Genesis of the U. S., v. 1, p. 479.

[53]Purchas: Pilgrimes, v. 4, p. 1753.

[54]As illustrative of such mistakes in diagnosis, W. A. Barber in the U. S. Health Reports, quotes Thayer to show that malaria is blamed for much illness of which it is not the cause. Thus, 4,407 deaths from malaria and 3,937 from typhoid were reported in New York, Brooklyn and Baltimore between 1883 and 1889, while in the Johns Hopkins Hospital covering the same period 48 deaths actually occurred from typhoid and only 3 from malaria. Obviously, the clinical diagnosis of malaria as late as 1889 was in the majority of cases incorrect.

"force her out to replanting of corn."[55]   Beverley, writing in the first part of the next century but evidently referring to the colony in the Seventeenth Century, said that "the first sickness that any newcomer happens to have there, he unfairly calls a seasoning, be it fever, ague or anything else . . . their intermitting fevers, as well as their agues, are very troublesome if a fit remedy be not applied; but of late the doctors there have made use of the cortex Peruviana with success."[56]

These five references to ague do not constitute enough evidence to warrant the statements of the historians.   It is true there were marshes and stagnant water about Jamestown.   Strachey noted that the town was "seated in somewhat an unwholesome and sickly ayre by reason it is in a marish ground, low, flat to the river."[57]   As early as the times of Homer malaria had been associated with stagnant marshes.   The Brahmanical Susruta in the Fifth Century ascribed malaria to mosquitoes.   There were probably any number of mosquitoes in the James River marshes, of the anopheles family, too.   A Henrico County inventory in 1684 includes "two peices of Mosquito Cloath."   Beverley describes the insects in detail: "Mosquitoes are a sort of vermin of less danger, but much more troublesome, because more frequent.   They are a long tailed gnat, such as are in all fens and low grounds in England, and I think have no

---

[55]Henrico County Records, v. 5, p. 36.
[56]Beverley: History of Virginia, ch. 20.
[57]Purchas: Pilgrimes, v. 4, p. 1753.

other difference from them than the name. Neither are they in Virginia troubled with them anywhere but in their low grounds and marshes. These insects, I believe, are stronger, and continue longer there, by reason of the warm sun, than in England. Whoever is persecuted with them in his house, may get rid of them by this easy remedy: let him set open his windows at sunset and shut them again before the twilight be quite shut in. All the mosquitoes in the room will go out at the windows and leave the room clear."[58]

Malaria undoubtedly occurred sporadically throughout the century. It may have assumed epidemic proportions at times. According to Heiser it was pandemic in 1657-59 and again in 1677-95. It was epidemic throughout the Seventeenth Century in England, and Willis, Morton, Sydenham and Lucas-Schact gave excellent descriptions of it. There is no evidence, however, that malaria was responsible for a preponderating part of the great mortalities of the Seventeenth Century in Virginia. No one doubts that there were marshes, mosquitoes and sickness along the James River, with probably the expected amount of malaria; but there is no record that it was of the pernicious and decimating type.

Besides the paucity of contemporary references there are other reasons for doubting the epidemic manifestations of malaria in Virginia in the early years. For example, there is no evidence that the American Indian had malaria before the coming of the white man, or that native mosquitoes were

---

[58]Beverley: History of Virginia, ch. 19.

infected with the plasmodium before 1607. Malaria, "the Kentish disorder" as it was often called, was common enough in England at the time, and the planters probably enjoyed as much natural immunity to the disease as did their fellows on the other side of the Atlantic. Furthermore, the fact that the high mortality in Virginia was chiefly among newcomers and that, once "seasoned," the colonists enjoyed good health, indicates that the fatal disease was more apt to have been typhoid, one attack of which confers immunity, than malaria, which is a disease prone to annual recurrence.

VIII

Winter Epidemics

Three times during this century there were epidemics occuring in the winter, attended by a fearful mortality. These were probably respiratory infections—influenza, pneumonia or pleurisy, all of which at times reach epidemic proportions. Nothing in the contemporary descriptions of the epidemics, however, warrants a positive opinion. There is this from Butler's accusation against the colony in 1623: "people are forced to a Continuall wadinge and wettinge of themselves and yt in ye prime of winter when ye Shipps commonly arrive, and therby get such vyolent surfetts of colde uppon colde as seldom leave them until they leave to live."[59] In the same year Mr. George Sandys writes to Mr. Ferrar in England, "Such a pestilent fever rageth this winter

---

[59]Neill: Virginia Company of London, pp. 395-401.

amongst us; never knowne before in Virginia, by the infected people that came over in ye Abigail, who were poisoned with stinkeinge beer all falling sick and many dying, everywhere dispersing the contagion."[60]   Discounting the obvious prejudice against the bad beer and bearing in mind Butler's complaint about this same winter, one concludes that the pestilent fever of the winter of 1623 was evidently respiratory.   DeVries is authority for the statement that during the winter of 1635 great mortality prevailed among the colonists.[61]   Memoranda concerning the House of Burgesses, 1685-91, include a note for April 1688: "A fast for ye great mortality (the first time the Winter distemper was soe very fatal . . . the people dyed, 1688, as in a plague . . . bleeding the remedy, Ld Howard had 80 ounces taken from him . . .)"[62]   There was a fresh outbreak of this epidemic the next winter.

In Europe during this century there were a number of recorded epidemics of respiratory diseases which the accompanying table summarizes.   Influenza was epidemic in New England in 1647 and again in 1697-99.[63]   Its greatest violence was in January, when whole families were sick at once and entire towns were seized at nearly the same time.   One Connecticut town buried seventy of its inhabitants in three months.   The records of our Virginia epidemics do not

---

[60]Brown: First Republic, p. 505.
[61]Neill: Virginia Carolorum, p. 128.
[62]Ludwell Papers, in Virginia Magazine of History and Biography, v. 5, p. 61.
[63]Packard: History of Medicine in the U. S.

INFLUENZA EPIDEMICS*

DATE	GENERAL FEATURES	ORIGIN	DIRECTION OF SPREAD	LOCALITIES AFFECTED
1593	Involved a wide area of Europe	Belgium— Extended over Europe	?	
1626	Local			Described in Italy
1627	In America		From North America to West Indies and Chili	
1647	In America (Webster)			
1658	Local	England?		England Treptow
1675	Over Western Europe	Germany?		Germany Hungary England France
1688	Apparently localized in Great Britain and Ireland	England		England Ireland
1693	England and Continent	Dublin		Dublin Oxford London Holland Flanders
1709 1712	Period of extensive epidemics	Germany?	From Germany to Holland and Italy	Italy France Belgium Germany Denmark

*An Epidemiologic Study by Warren T. Vaughan, M. D.
(Condensed and modified)

coincide with either of these New England outbreaks. According to the table, influenza is said to have been localized in Great Britain and Ireland in 1688, but the fast for "ye great mortality" that same winter in Virginia indicates that the disease had spread to the colony.

IX

Plague

Was Seventeenth Century Virginia ever afflicted with the plague? Gabriel Archer in 1609 mentions that one of the ships, the *Vice-Admiral,* "was said to have the plague in her."[64] Four of the London Company's fleet in 1609 were reported to be infected with calenture and the London plague, and from sixty to ninety of their passengers died at sea.[65] Later on in the century we find an isolated reference to plague in the Northampton County records: "John Stringer chirurgeon hath given his attendance upon Rich. Newport, Gent." and also upon Edward Newport, both of whom had died of "a contagious disease called the Plague."[66]

There is scant evidence for the presence of plague in colonial Virginia. Packard does not mention it as having been present in America in the Seventeenth Century. On the other hand the city of London was repeatedly visited by plague between 1603 and 1611. Between March and

[64]Brown: Genesis of the U. S., v. 1, p. 329.
[65]Brown: First Republic, p. 97.
[66]Northampton County Records, v. 1640-45, pp. 218-219.

December 1603, 30,561 died of it. From December 1605 to January 1607 (five days after Newport sailed for Virginia) 2,124 victims were buried in London.[67] It was thought that the surplus population of England was the cause of the plague, and this is often assigned as one of the objects of colonization. A letter from the Council and Company of the Honorable Plantation in Virginia to the Lord Mayor, Aldermen and Companies of London, dated 1609, says: "Desirous to ease the cities and suburbs of a swarm of unnecessary inmates as a continual cause of dearth and famine, and the very original cause of all the plagues that happen in this Kingdom, have advised . . . their remove into this Plantation of Virginia."[68] That the Virginia colonists had plague at least on their minds is shown in the "Articles, Laws and Orders, Divine Politique and Martial for the colony in Virginia," which were "exemplified and approved" June 22, 1610.[69] A severe penalty was attached to throwing soap suds in the open street, because in London it was thought that "Not only soap boilers and vendors of it but all the washer-women and all they whose business it was to use soap—nay, they who only wore shirts washed with soap—presently died of the plague."[70] The evidence for plague is probably as great as the evidence for yellow fever or malaria. Certainly in the rat infested ships of those

[67]Brown: First Republic, p. 13.
[68]Brown: Genesis of the U. S., v. 1, p. 252.
[69]Brown: First Republic, p. 131.
[70]Ibid.

days, with the plague raging in London, there was every
opportunity to pass on the infection to the colony.

X

Smallpox

Smallpox, unknown in America until after the advent of
the Spaniards, was first recorded in the West Indies in 1507.
Africa had long been an endemic center of smallpox, and
the importation of slaves from Africa was often followed
by an outbreak of the disease.   No early epidemics are
recorded in this country, though a disease which was common in England undoubtedly affected the colonists as well.
In a population unprotected by vaccination smallpox eventually attacked practically every one, and there were few
adults who did not bear evidence of this with a pitted face.
Royalty was no exception.   But, as in the case of the other
exanthemata, it was chiefly the children who were suscept-
ible.   They represented the non-immunes in the population,
and the periodic epidemics which occurred among them were
spaced about a generation apart.   The scarcity of children
among the early settlers and the undoubted predominance
of immunized adults accounts for the low incidence of smallpox in the first half of the first century in Virginia.

The first recorded epidemic in the colony occurred in
1667.[71]   In that year a sailor with smallpox landed at
Accomack. He was isolated by the chirurgeons but escaped

---

[71]Wise: Eastern Shore, p. 63.   Packard records the first outbreak in
New Netherlands in 1663 and in New England in 1666.

to a nearby Indian town and infected two tribes. The disease spread all over the Eastern Shore with fearful mortality. During the epidemic the "Colonel and Commander" of Northampton County, acting in his capacity of health officer, issued a proclamation warning all families affected with smallpox to allow no member "to go forth their doors until their full cleansing, that is to say, thirtie dayes after their receiving the sd smallpox, least the sd disease shoulde spreade by infection like the plague of leprosy . . . such as shall no-things notice of this premonition and charge, but beast like shall p'sume to act and doe contrarily, may expect to be severely punished according to the Statute of King James in such case provided for their contempt herein; God save the King."[72]

In 1696 smallpox was so prevalent at Jamestown that the Assembly asked for a recess, declaring that the disease was known to be very fatal and was rapidly propagated, especially during a session of the house which necessarily brought a large crowd to Jamestown and exposed them to the disease.[73]

XI

Measles

Packard does not mention measles as epidemic in this country until 1713, but the Virginia colony was sorely affected in the last decade of the preceding century. A "Proc-

[72]Bruce: Institutional History of Virginia, v. 2, p. 18.
[73]Ibid., v. 2, p. 488.

lamation appointing a Day of Humiliation and Prayer"
was signed by Governor Andros after the members of the
Council had resolved that "It haveing pleased Almighty
God to Afflict this Country with the measles whereof Severall have dyed, It is the opinion and Advice of the Councill
that Wednesday the 17th of May next [1693] be set apart
throughout this Colony, humbly to Implore by fasting and
Prayers, the Mercy of Almighty God in the pardon and for-
giveness of our Sins. . . ."[74] Since measles and smallpox
were often confused, this epidemic may have been the
latter.[75]

Other epidemical diseases such as scarlet fever, diph-
theria and hydrophobia, which occurred elsewhere in America during this century, are not mentioned in the early Virginia records.

XII

Fluxes and Fevers

The "Flixes" of Percy and the "Bloody Flux" of other
contemporary writers were terms in vogue in England at the
time, and were used synonymously with dysentery. Dysentery, as is well known, is an acute intestinal disease characterized by fever, diarrhea, cramps and bloody mucous
evacuations. Many attacks of dysentery are milder and

74Executive Journals, Council of Colonial Virginia, v. 1, pp. 285, 292.
75The first medical book published in America dealt with smallpox,
and was entitled "Brief Rule to Guide the Common People of New
England how to order themselves in the Smallpox or Measles," by
Thomas Thatcher, clergyman and M. D., 1677.

show no blood and mucus. The mortality varies from twelve to twenty-five percent. Typhoid fever is a disease often associated with diarrhea and bloody stools, and undoubtedly cases of it were classified under the general heading of "flux."

Lord Delaware, who was himself a catalogue of Seventeenth Century diseases, complained that among other ailments "the Flux surprised me, and kept me many daiès; then the cramp assaulted my weak body, with strong paines . . . & afterwards the Gout . . . afflicted me. . . ."[76] Percy, speaking of the diseases of 1607 and 1608, mentions "Flixes" among the serious disorders of the first years. In 1618 the *Neptune* and the *Treasurer* were said to have "brought a most pestilent disease (called the bloody flux) which infected almost the whole colony. That disease, notwithstanding all our former afflictions, was never known before amongst us."[77] Evidently there was something new in this type of flux, either the fact that it was bloody, or that it had a high mortality, or that it was brought in by the ships. Undoubtedly these fluxes, introduced in 1618, were prevalent in 1619 also, and may have been responsible in part for the adjournment of the first House of Burgesses. The session came to an abrupt end on the fourth of August 1619, "being constrained by the intemperature of the weather and the falling sick of diverse of the Burgesses to breake up

---

[76]Brown: Genesis of the U. S., v. 1, p. 479.
[77]Brown: First Republic, p. 282.

so abruptly. . . ."[78]   One of the members, Mr. Shelly, died during the session, and the Speaker himself was laid low. The excessive heat of August was said to have been a factor in producing the sickness.   That the sickness of this year was alarming is shown in a public letter from the Governor, which reached England in February 1620 in the *Diana*, along with the journal of the first General Assembly.   He asked for physicians and apothecaries and told of the sickness, which he attributed to the colonists' having to eat pork, fresh and unseasoned for want of salt.   He asked that Sir Thomas Dale's salt works, which had been allowed to go to ruin, be set up again.[79]   In modern phraseology, the Governor was attributing the sickness to a food poisoning. A somewhat similar explanation of the flux which occurred the following year was given in the Company's letter of August 1621: "And here we cannot hide from you an information that is lately given us that sutch provisions as we send with new men were taken from them and Indian corn given them instead thereof, the extreme labour of beating thereof being no small disheartening to the new comers and the suddaine change of dyett is affirmed confidently to be the cause of the flux in our men to an irreparable loss."[80]   This reminds one of the Indian corn feasts which were held yearly and which had a medico-religious significance.   Gorging with

---

[78]Proceedings of the first General Assembly of Virginia, printed in Colonial Records of Virginia.

[79]Brown: First Republic, p. 327.

[80]Neill: Virginia Company of London, p. 237.

green corn produced violent diarrhea among the Indians and was considered a valuable annual purge.

That these intestinal disorders were connected with food and drink is further borne out in the statement of Strachey, who in 1610 wisely observed that the Jamestown water supply, "a well sixe or seven fathom deepe, fed by the brackish River owzing into it," was one of the chief causes "of many diseases and sicknesses which have happened to our people, who are indeede strangely afflicted with Fluxes. . ."[81] It is not unreasonable to suppose that typhoid also lurked in the shallow Jamestown well, and some of the bloody flux was undoubtedly of this origin. Sir Francis Wyatt describes what was almost certainly typhoid in a letter written at Jamestown during his term as Governor: "There are no Leveres [Livers] here: no where better stomacks, nor sounder sleepes: But certaine it is new comers seldome passe July and August without a burning fever, which thorough intemperate drinking of water often drawes after it the flixe or dropsy, and where many are sick together, is infectious: This requires a skilful Phisitian, convenient diett and lodging with diligent attendance, few dying of the first brunt of sickness, but upon relapses for want of strengthening diett and good drinke to repaire the losse of that bloud, which is taken from them. . . ."[82]

The Reverend John Clayton, minister at Jamestown 1684-86, shows great alarm in a letter, probably written

---

[81]Purchas: Pilgrimes, v. 4, p. 1753.
[82]William and Mary Quarterly, second series, v. 6, p. 117.

to Dr. Boyle, over "the Distemper of the Colick that is predominant and has miserable sad effects it begins with violent gripes wch declining takes away the use of limbs. Their fingers stand stiffly bent, the hands of some hang as if they were loose at the wrists from the arms, they are sceletons so meagre & leane that a consumption might seeme a fatning to them, cruelly are they distracted wth a flatus, & at length those that seemeingly recover are oft troubled wth a sort of gout."[83]   This does not sound like any of the intestinal disorders, but fits in very well with the description of lead colic.   The sources of lead might have been leaden containers of drinking water, wine or cider.   In 1572 there was an epidemic of lead colic in southern France, probably due to the lead in cider and wine presses.   In the Eighteenth Century Sir George Baker showed that "Devonshire Colic" was definitely due to the lead used in the vats and cider presses of Devon.   In 1757 Théodore Tronchin showed that colic was produced by water passed through gutters from leaden roofs; and in 1725 Thomas Cadwalader of Philadelphia wrote an *Essay on the West-India Dry-Gripes,* which was printed by Benjamin Franklin, and which proved that that disease was caused by rum distilled through lead pipes.

Beverley, writing at the beginning of the next century, refers to "Fluxes, fevers and the bellyache" and relates them to improper eating.   Dysentery, therefore, must have been

---

[83]William and Mary Quarterly, second series, v. 1, p. 114.

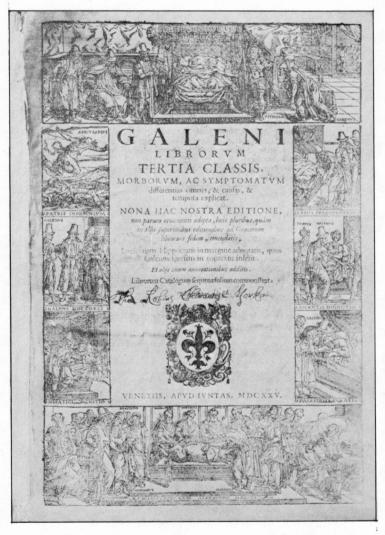

Title page of the copy of Galen's *Opera* owned in the Seventeenth
Century by Dr. Thomas Robins, of York County.

a rather common summertime complaint in Seventeenth Century Virginia. It was probably more prevalent and virulent when the colonists were crowded into such palisaded towns as Jamestown, Henrico and Kecoughtan.

Not until the discovery of the bacterial cause of most of the fevers (1880) was there any real understanding of these very common disorders, although some advance had been made over the Hippocratic division into intermittent and continued fevers. Rhazes in the Ninth Century separated smallpox from measles. Sydenham recognized scarlet fever and wrote extensively on continued and intermittent fever and on smallpox. Louis (1819) and Gerhard (1832) placed typhoid and typhus in classes by themselves. As late as 1842 Bartlett, writing on fevers in the United States, classified them all under four headings: typhus, typhoid, periodic and yellow fever. It is clear that great confusion and ignorance characterized our conception of the fevers prior to the last decade of the Nineteenth Century.

During the latter half of the Seventeenth Century the therapeutic effect of cinchona bark was of great value in differentiating the fevers, but it was 1640 before it was introduced into Europe and 1676 before Sydenham was enthusiastically recommending it—hardly time for it to affect colonial practice in that century. The term fever, then, as applied to Seventeenth Century diseases by writers of that day was an inclusive word which might have signified any of a number of fevers as we now classify them. The most distinguished English physician of the century said in

1666 that two-thirds of medical practice dealt with fevers; yet outside of smallpox, measles and scarletina he was compelled to throw them all into the two great groups of continuous and intermittent. The "burning fevers" of Jamestown in 1607 were hardly smallpox, measles or scarlet fever. Writers who called diseases by their outstanding symptoms ("swellings" for beriberi, and "bloody flux" for dysentery) would have used more descriptive terms for the eruptive fevers. They were thoroughly familiar with the intermittent fevers (malaria) of England, and the ague which so well describes them was a word they would likewise have used had malaria been the chief cause of the "burning fevers."

It seems likely, then, that Percy was describing a continuous fever—a disease characterized by an unremitting diurnal monotony. No disease fits this description so well as the typhoid-paratyphoid infections. Malaria, starvation fever and other febrile diseases may have occurred, but the burning fever of 1607 is more apt to have been typhoid than any other. Though not differentiated clinically until 1819 the ravages of typhoid are plainly seen in historical references to undoubted epidemics. Sudhoff, the greatest of medical historians, holds that the Neopolitan Epidemic of 1495-96 was an outbreak of typhoid or paratyphoid infection, against the older opinion that it was syphilis brought back by the soldiers of Columbus. According to G. Stecker there was a camp epidemic of typhoid at Louvain and Nimwegen in 1635, and Thomas Willis in 1643 described it among Parliamentary troops. The prevalence of typhoid in Europe, the probable presence of carriers among the adventurers to Virginia, the crowded, insanitary arrangements on ships and at Jamestown make typhoid a very likely cause of the fevers and the high death rate among our early settlers. Some of the "fevers" so frequently referred to by the early writers may have been malaria, dysentery or influenza, but typhoid, which is a disease of the summer season, must have accounted for much of the dreaded summer sickness and probably killed off more than all the others combined.

XIII

Calenture and Yellow Fever

Calenture is defined as a delirious fever believed to attack mariners in the tropics, often causing hallucinations which make the victim plunge into the sea. The word is used by Berenger-Feraud as one of the synonyms for yellow fever, and lay writers of Virginia history have used it similarly.

Captain John Radcliffe writes to the Earl of Salisbury from Jamestown, October 4, 1609, "Sir Thomas Gates and Sir George Summers Captaine Newport and 180 persons or ther about are not yet arrived. . . . The other Shipps came all in, but not together; we were thus separated by a storme, two shipps had great loss of men by the Calenture and most of them all much weather beaten."[84] In the same

---

[84]Brown: Genesis of the U. S., v. 1, p. 334.

year Gabriel Archer writes, "We ran a Southerly course
from the Tropicke of Cancer . . . so that by the fervent heat
and loomes breezes, many of our men fell sicke of the
Calenture, and out of two ships was throwne over-boord
thirtie-two persons."[85]   Brown, commenting upon the calenture ships and the mortality at Jamestown which followed
their arrival, says, "Early in December (1609) the remnant
of 'Sir Thomas Gates his fleet,' reached England, with Captain John Smith and full reports showing conclusively that
the colony had been found in most deplorable condition in
August, 1609, and had been left . . . with a terrible disease
(the yellow fever, or London plague, or both) raging at
Jamestown."[86]

A *Brief Declaration* by the planters, written in 1624,
states that within a few months after Lord Delaware's
arrival not less than a hundred and fifty died of calenture
and fever.[87]   The only other reference we have been able
to find in this century occurs in Bullock's *Virginia impartially
Examined,* published in 1649.   Here the author remarks
that "in June, July and August . . . the poore Servant goes
daily through the rowes of Tobacco . . . and being overheated he is struck with a Calenture or Feaver and so
perisheth. . . ."[88]

Yellow fever is a disease about the origin of which the

---

[85]Brown: Genesis of the U. S., v. 1, p. 329.
[86]Brown: First Republic, p. 105.
[87]Calendar British State Papers, v. 1574-1660, p. 67.
[88]Bullock: Virginia impartially Examined, p. 11.

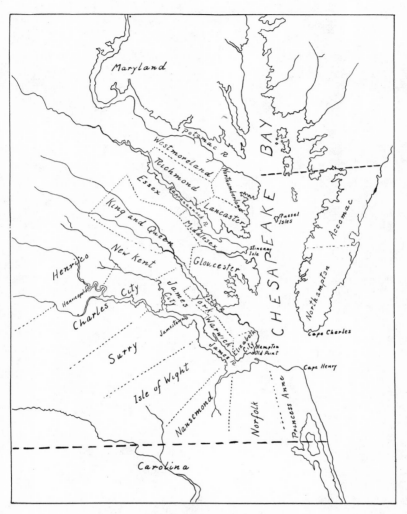

A map of Seventeenth Century Virginia.

best opinion has for many years differed. It is usually stated that the white man first came in contact with it in the West Indies in 1495 and that infected ships spread the disease to the mainland of America. This is the view held by Berenger-Feraud. The late Dr. Henry R. Carter believed that yellow fever originated on the west coast of Africa and spread to this country with the slave trade, borne by mosquitoes (stegomyia) and not by infected persons.[89] Epidemics are known to have occurred in Africa in the Sixteenth Century, and one is recorded in 1639. Yellow fever is essentially a disease of the tropics and sub-tropics, and its spread is intimately associated with the intermediate host, the *stegomyia fasciata*. The blood of the yellow fever patient is said not to be infectious for the mosquito after three days. Yellow fever is an acute disease, and cases of it developing soon after leaving port, whether it were Africa or the West Indies, would have terminated favorably or otherwise before reaching America in the slow sailing vessels of the Seventeenth Century. How, then, was it possible for this disease to be conveyed from either the Antilles or Africa to the coast of Virginia? The only tenable explanation is that in the open water buckets, common on the ships of those days, the *stegomyia fasciata* propagated, continued the infection on ship board, and in the new world survived long enough to spread the contagion.

The early proven epidemics in America were in the sea-

---

[89]Personal communication from Dr. Carter's daughter.

port towns of New York, 1668, Boston, 1691, and Charleston, 1699. In the Philadelphia epidemic Benjamin Rush noted that the infected part of the city was that part around the water fronts, just where the *stegomyia fasciata* took up its abode after leaving the ship and so spread the infection. In the same way yellow fever came to Virginia, in the bodies of imported mosquitoes. Even today, about Norfolk and Portsmouth, mosquito surveys show the presence of a few *stegomyia fasciata.*

Although yellow fever did occur epidemically in the Eighteenth Century and classical studies of it were made by John Mitchell, its presence in the Seventeenth Century in Virginia is extremely doubtful. It is usually stated that yellow fever did not appear in America until 1647. It was at this time that the great epidemic occurred in Cuba, and the first outbreak in America is recorded as the "Barbadoes Distemper."

The facts appear to be that endemic centers of yellow fever undoubtedly existed on the west coast of Africa and in the Antilles, and trading vessels from these places not infrequently touched on the Virginia coast. It is possible that these vessels may have conveyed infected mosquitoes to North America. A disease called calenture occurred upon some of these ships in 1609, and subsequent to their arrival in Virginia epidemic diseases were raging at Jamestown. In 1610 the disease is again mentioned. The reference in 1648 is less convincing. It is possible that yellow fever did occur in Virginia in the Seventeenth Century. It is a curious fact, however, that the references to calenture occur only in the first year or two of the colony's life and that with increasing trade and commerce there were no further outbreaks. In the next century, when undoubted yellow fever did occur, the outbreaks were increasingly frequent until the quarantine of 1856. In other words, with a growing commerce, once the specific mosquito was certainly introduced we should expect what actually occurred, increasing outbreaks of the disease. As this was not the case in the Seventeenth Century, doubt is cast upon the existence of the infection at all.

YELLOW FEVER EPIDEMICS IN THE 17TH CENTURY[90]

1520 Africa
1553 Africa
1558 Africa
1588 Africa
1599 Africa
1635 Lesser Antilles
1639 Africa
1640 Lesser Antilles and South America
1643 South America
1645 Lesser Antilles
1647 Lesser Antilles and South America
1648 Lesser and Greater Antilles

[90]*Traité Théorique et Clinique de la Fièvre Jaune*, by L. J. B. Berenger-Feraud.

1649 Greater Antilles
1652 Lesser Antilles
1655 Greater Antilles
1656 Lesser and Greater Antilles
1665 Lesser Antilles
1668 Lesser and Greater Antilles, North America and South America
1694 Lesser Antilles, South America and Europe
1695 Lesser Antilles and North America
1696 Lesser and Greater Antilles, Central America and Europe
1697 Lesser and Greater Antilles, North America and South America
1698 Lesser Antilles
1699 Lesser and Greater Antilles, Central America and North America

XIV
Sanitation

Compared with modern ideas of sanitation and hygiene, Seventeenth Century notions seem very crude. Yet one cannot read the contemporary writings of this century without being impressed with the fact that there did exist some wholesome ideas about the causation and prevention of disease. One sees this in the current disapproval of poor food, crowded quarters, foul ships, marshy land, stagnant drinking water, and in the recognition of contagion and the need for quarantine.

The earliest record of quarantine is of that put into effect by Lord Delaware at Kecoughtan.[91] The smallpox epidemic of 1667 might have been prevented had not the quarantine instituted by the chirurgeons of Accomac been broken by an incorrigible sailor. The martial law established by Sir Thomas Gates in 1610 and enlarged and approved by Lord Delaware in 1611 takes account of foul waters in the street, the possibility of contaminating the drinking water, and the necessity for placing latrines at a safe distance from the wells: "There shall no man or woman, Launderer or Launderesse, dare to wash uncleane linnen, drive bucks, or throw out the water or suds of fowle cloathes, in the open streete, within the Pallizadoes, or within forty foote of the same, nor rench, and make cleane, any kettle, pot, or pan, or such like vessell within twenty foote of the olde well, or new Pumpe: nor shall any one aforesaid, within lesse then a quarter of one mile from the Pallizadoes, dare to doe the necessities of nature, since by these unmanly, slothfull, and loathsome immodesties, the whole Fort may be choaked, and poisoned with ill aires, and so corrupt (as in all reason cannot but much infect the same) and this shall they take notice of, and avoide, upon paine of whipping and further punishment, as shall be thought meete, by the censure of a martiall Court."[92]

The provision for raising the bedstead at least three feet from the ground was dictated by a fear of dampness:

---

[91] Cridlin: History of Virginia.
[92] Force: Tracts, v. 3, "Lawes Divine, Morall & Martiall . . .," p. 15.

"Every man shall have an especiall and due care, to keepe his house sweete and cleane, as also so much of the streete as lieth before his door, and especially he shall so provide, and set his bedstead whereon he lieth, that it may stand three foote at lease from the ground, as he will answere the contrarie at a martiall Court."[93]

Military sanitation took cognizance of the importance of cleanliness, diet and proper sleeping quarters, and is embodied in instructions such as the following: "Hee [the Lieutenant] is amongst other his duties most carefully, like a charitable and wel instructed Christian, mercifull and compassionate, make often and daily survey of such of his company as shalbe visited with sicknesse, or wounded by any casualty of warre, gunpoulder, or other-wise, in which hee shall take such order that the lodgings of such as shalbe so sicke or hurt, be sweet and cleanely kept, them-selves attended and drest, and to the uttermost of his power to procure, either from the store, or Phisition and Surgeons chest, such comforts, healps and remedies, as may be administred and applied unto them, and to have a care that they be not defrauded of those meanes and remedies which are for them delivered out of the said store or chests. . . ."[94]

Reviewing the epidemics and mortality of this century in Virginia, one is impressed with the early decimating outbreaks of disease which allowed of practically no growth in population before 1630. Among the causes of mortality

---

[93]Force: Tracts, v. 3, "Lawes Divine, etc.," p. 16.
[94]Ibid., p. 47.

were famine, beriberi, scurvy, typhoid and dysentery; perhaps plague, yellow fever and malaria. After 1630 there was a gradual increase in population, but it was very slow considering the fact that 100,000 immigrated. Epidemic diseases which later beset the colony were influenza, pneumonia, perhaps pleurisy; lead poisoning, smallpox and measles. As the colony grew older it was less and less concentrated into a few towns along the rivers. The yearly increment from immigration, compared to the fixed population, was less. Food became more plentiful, Indians a less serious menace, more children were born and lived. All of these factors were reflected in the changing mortality rates and the prevailing epidemic diseases.

CHAPTER III

MEDICAL EDUCATION

I

HE first doctors to practice in Virginia were picked and sent over by the London Company. They were English physicians transferred to Virginia soil. Their medical education was obtained like that of other English physicians of that day.

Birth often determined the choice of a profession. "When there were three or four sons to be provided for by a father who was a country gentleman, it was usual, in the seventeenth century, to keep the eldest at home if he was to inherit the whole of the landed estates; the second son was sent to one of the great universities, in order to prepare himself to enter a learned profession, such as law, physic or divinity; the third was apprenticed to a local solicitor, apothecary, or surgeon; the fourth to a pewterer or watchmaker, or the like. It will be observed that the employments selected were graduated in social importance according to the relative ages of the sons."[1] Oxford and Cambridge offered courses in medicine. Better opportunities for study, however, were to be had on the Continent, especially

---

[1]Bruce: Social Life in Virginia in the 17th Century, p. 83.

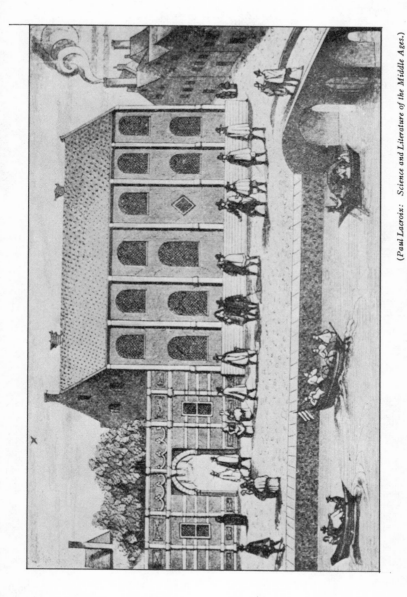

(*Paul Lacroix: Science and Literature of the Middle Ages.*)

The University of Leyden, from which Dr. Bohun and other Virginia physicians were
probably graduated.

in Italy and France. The mediaeval texts, Hippocrates, Dioscorides, Galen and Avicenna, though still revered, were now augmented by better and newer works. Garrison says of the medical education of Giles Firmin, who was lecturing on anatomy in New England before 1647, "His anatomy he got from Vesalius, Paré, Fallopius, and Spigelius; his internal medicine was a mixture of the Greeks, Fernelius, Van Helmont, and Sir Kenelm Digby; his pathology was mythology."

As the student of the preceding century had been stimulated by the widespread interest in anatomy and botany, so the would-be doctor of the Seventeenth must have been influenced by the soundings then under way in the new sciences of chemistry and physics. He had no real bedside instruction, though a few gestures had been made in this direction. Pathology was in swaddling clothes, waiting for the popular prejudice against autopsies to die out. In England anatomical teaching must have been dry indeed, for it was mostly out of the books. Edinburgh, which took the lead among the English schools, did not have a skeleton until 1697.

In Munk's Roll of the Royal College of Physicians from 1570-1700 the names of 642 physicians are listed. Although these were the most distinguished physicians of that period, 167 had no degree in medicine, though they often had other academic degrees. Four hundred and seventy-three held doctors' degrees in medicine, and two were bachelors in medicine. Of these 475 doctors, 131 received their medical education at Cambridge, 86 at Oxford, 69 at Padua, 64 at Leyden, 21 at Utrecht, 12 at Montpellier, 11 at Caen, and 8 at Basle. A sprinkling of other universities makes up the rest. Of course the great majority of English physicians had had no university training. They were the ordinary physicians, trained by apprenticeship; the chirurgeons, products sometimes of the Barbers' College; the bone-setters, and others bordering on quackery.

Against this background we must view the medical education of our Seventeenth Century Virginia physicians. Some of the earlier ones had doubtless touched elbows with Harvey at Padua under the tutelage of Fabricius of Aquapendente; or at Leyden had studied under Sylvius, Ruysch, Nuck or Bidloo; or at Montpellier under Barbeirac. Others got no farther than Sydenham, who was kept out of the College of Physicians because he did not have the M. D. degree. The majority must have entered medicine through apprenticeships, no mean way of acquiring medical knowledge in those days, and one of which Edward Jenner was an illustrious example in the next century.

II

Most of the Virginians referred to in the colonial records as "doctor" probably had no academic right to such a title. Yet a few undoubtedly did hold degrees in medicine. The earliest of these were Dr. Walter Russell (1608), "Doctour of Physicke," and Laurence Bohun (1610), "Docktor in phisick." Bohun probably received his degree at Leyden, for he was said to have studied "among the most learned Surgeons and Physitions in the Netherlands." He was succeeded by John Pott in 1621. Dr. Gulstone had recommended "Mr. Pottes a master of arts . . . well practiced in chirurgery and physicke." While clearly a man of education and experience, Pott had evidently not attained to the M. D. degree, though he was often referred to as "doctor." Of the physicians known to have practised in Virginia under the Company prior to 1624 probably none except Dr. Russell and Dr. Bohun held a degree in medicine.

In spite of the popular confusion of titles the value of a university education was sufficiently understood to serve as the basis of the discrimination in the Virginia fee bill of 1736 in favor of the man of education. We know of just one Virginia doctor of the latter half of the century who had a degree—John Lee, Bachelor of Arts of Queen's College about 1658, and later Doctor of Physick.[2] Others there undoubtedly were, because the custom was common, among the well-to-do, of sending their children to England for higher education. Michel observed that "it was customary for wealthy parents . . . to send their sons to England to study there. But experience showed that not many of them came back. Most of them died of smallpox, to which sickness the children of the West are subject."[3]

---

[2] Bruce: Institutional History of Virginia, v. 1, p. 318.
[3] Virginia Magazine of History and Biography, v. 24, "Journey of Michel to Va."

There were easier and quicker roads to medicine than through the universities. Some Virginians must have studied under eminent doctors in England. Dr. John Woodall, a famous English surgeon of the first half of the century, writes to Virginia to his "loveing friend Mr. Wake, Surgeone." Wake had probably studied under Woodall in London.

At a time when the passage to England was both difficult and expensive, the greater number of Virginia doctors naturally received all of their education at home. Education had received serious and often elaborate attention since the early days of the colony. The Company had planned to establish a university and a free school at the present site of Dutch Gap, and today a monument stands there to commemorate the project. There was to have been also a college for the Indians—a venture which attracted magnificent gifts from England. The funds were invested in the iron industry at Falling Creek and were wiped out with the annihilation of that plant in the massacre of 1622.

In 1634, through the gift of Benjamin Symmes, a free school for the children of the parishes of Elizabeth City and Kecoughtan was established. It had "200 acres of land. A fine house upon it. Forty milch kine and other accomodations." In 1652 and 1659 similar schools were set up in Northumberland and Northampton Counties. Besides these there was Captain Moore's school in 1655, Richard Russell's school in 1667, and Mr. King's school in 1669. In 1686 two persons were appointed in each county to examine and approve school masters. Yet Governor Berkeley declared in 1671, "I thank God there are no free schools nor printing" in Virginia. He doubtless meant that there were none like the free schools of New England. The dream of higher education in the colony was not realized until 1693, when Dr. Blair arrived from England with a charter for William and Mary College.

The preliminary education of Virginians planning the practice of medicine was acquired in these free schools, which several physicians played a part in establishing. In 1634 Dr. Thomas Eaton acquired a patent for two hundred acres of land in Elizabeth City County and founded a free school for children of that county. The original endowment was "five hundred acres of improved land, two negroes, twelve cows, two bulls and twenty hogs, with a substantial residence and large quantity of household furniture."[4] It taught "English and Grammar." The school was incorporated with the Symmes Free School in 1805 and named Hampton Academy. As late as 1902 part of the original endowment was used to erect the Symmes-Eaton Academy, which is now part of the Virginia public school system. In 1697 Dr. George Eland, a physician by profession, was appointed master of the Eaton School.[5]

In 1686 Nathaniel Hill, physician and school master, moved from Gloucester to Henrico. According to the court record, "Upon his petition it is order'd (for ye encourage-

---

[4]Bruce: Institutional History of Virginia, v. 1, pp. 353-56.
[5]Ibid., v. 1, p. 355.

ment of Learning and instruction of Youth in this county by inviting able tutors here to reside) that he be this year free and exempted from paying any levies."[6]

School masters in New Amsterdam also practised medicine. There was Adam Rolansten, who "was expected to supplement the work of the dominie by acting as a worthy consoler of the sick by promoting religious worship in the capacities of precentor and church clerk and by turning the hour glass to indicate to the preacher that the time allotted for his sermon had elapsed."[7]

III

Indentured servitude prevailed in all the colonies in the Seventeenth and Eighteenth Centuries and had little competition from African slavery before 1700. From 1607 to 1619 all the Virginia planters were servants of the Company. The number of "indented" servants increased rapidly between 1619 and 1675. In the later years of the century an average of 6,000 was maintained in the colony. On the whole they were well treated, often mingled socially with their masters, and obtained positions of prominence in the community when they became freedmen.[8] They came from England, Wales, Scotland and Ireland, some voluntarily, some involuntarily. In general they were a wholesome in-

---

[6]Henrico County Records, v. 2, p. 213.
[7]Colton: Annals of Old Manhattan.
[8]Ballagh: White Servitude in the Colony of Virginia. Bruce: Institutional History of Virginia.

fluence in the colony. Many were educated and belonged to the professions.

This system of indenture touched medicine in several particulars. In the next century the illness and threatened death of a slave was a serious matter, and masters saw to it that they had the best medical care. Under indentured servitude, where the term of indenture rarely exceeded five years, the master's risk was less, but he seems often to have realized that it was not good business to allow a sick servant to remain unattended. Chirurgeon Thomas Bunn in 1624 had three or four of Mr. Procter's servants under treatment in his own house at one time.[9] In 1682 "Samuel Rossier abt: thirty six years or thereabouts Deposeth . . . that [he] did hire a Made servt . . . for four years upon Consideration of the cure of her head . . . her head being very bad. She hath been wth me neare a twelve months and notwithstanding my careful endeavour and the costs of abt four hundred pounds of Tobo: and is not yet cured nor p'fectly well. . . ." Rossier's wife also testified that the servant had "an exceeding sore head" and that "her head hath cost me and my husband about 400 lb. tob."[10] Where masters grossly neglected their sick servants, the courts appear to have come to the rescue. In 1682 John Hall, servant of George Hambleton, "being lame & in a miserable condition," tells the court that his master "hath taken no care for ye cure thereof altho required by a former Court."

---

[9]Minutes of Council and General Court, p. 24.
[10]York County Records, v. 6, p. 430.

The court orders that Hambleton "take care to see ye same perfectly cured" and give bond "to defend ye parish of York harmlesse from what damage they may sustain."[11]

Many physicians were undoubtedly at one time indentured servants. Patrick Napier and Francis Haddon are known to have come to Virginia under terms of indenture, paying their passage money by a period of servitude.[12] John Williams was a Dutchman and a chirurgeon who was punished in 1640 for an attempted runaway while serving an indenture. John Inman is another example. In 1628 the Court orders "that John Inman Surgeon in Reguard hee came over wth the servants of Mr. Edw Bennett (as himselfe Confesseth) who paide for his passage shall remaine and serve uppon the plantacon of the said Mr. Edw Bennett untill he can procure testimony out of England to free himselfe."[13]

The more common type of indenture was the apprenticeship of a young man to an established physician to learn his profession. As there were no medical schools in America until 1776, this was the usual method of becoming a doctor. The earliest and most notable example in Virginia was that of Richard Townshend, who was apprenticed to Dr. Pott and who went to court in 1621 because his master had neglected his instruction. John Tilney probably served an apprenticeship to Dr. Holloway. His name appears in a

---

[11]York County Records, v. 6, p. 412.
[12]Greer: Early Virginia Immigrants. York County Records, v. 3, p. 214.
[13]Minutes of Council and General Court, p. 188.

Pharmacopœia Londinensis;

Rob. OR, THE *Knight*

London Dispensatory

FURTHER

Adorned by the *STUDIES* and

Collections of the *Fellows* now living, of the said *COLLEDGE.*

In this Impreſſion you may find,

1. Three hundred uſeful Additions.

2. All the Notes that were in the Margent are brought into the Book between two ſuch Crotchets as theſe [ ]

3. The Vertues, Qualities, and Properties of every *Simple.*

4. The Vertues and uſe of the *Compounds.*

5. Cautions in giving all Medicines that are dangerous.

6. All the Medicines that were in the *Old Latin Diſpenſa-tory,* and are left out in the *New Latin* one, are printed in this Impreſſion in Engliſh, with their Vertues.

7. A *KEY* to *Galen* and *Hippocrates* their *Method* of *Phy-ſick,* containing Thirty three Chapters.

8. In this Impreſſion, the *Latin* name of every one of the Compounds is printed, and in what Page of the new Fo-lio *Latin* Book they are to be found.

By *Nich. Culpeper* Gent. Student in Phyſick and Aſtrology.

London, Printed for *George Sawbridge,* at the Bible on *Ludgate-Hill.* 1675.

(Library of the Richmond Academy of Medicine, Miller Collection.)

Title page of Culpeper's *London Dispensatory,* a book often found in Seventeenth Century Virginia libraries.

list of persons imported by Holloway, and when the doctor
died in 1643 he bequeathed to John Tilney all his chirurgical
treatises and his medicine chest, instruments and lancets.[14]

Dr. Holloway had another apprentice, Gabriell Searle,
whom he had bought from William Holmes with the understanding that he was to educate him in the "art of chirurgery." The case was brought into the Northampton
Courts in 1643 on a complaint similar to that of Townshend
against Dr. Pott. A witness swore that he had heard Dr.
Holloway say "he would keep the boy Gabriell wch hee
bought of Mr. Holmes until he had a month to s've and
then hee the sd Holloway sayde hee would instruct and
shew him the sd Gabriell his trade." The jury found that
Holloway had "instructed him to the boyes best capacities in
the misticall arte of Chirurgery."[15] The Doctor died soon
after and bequeathed to Gabriell Searle "one heifer and
calf." The charge was frequently brought that the master
put his young apprentice to work at the most menial occupations and gave very little attention to his instruction in medicine. In Dr. Holloway's case the boy testified that his master "did not deny att any tyme to show him the Art of
Chirurgery."

An interesting contract between Charles Clay and Stephen
Tickner, chirurgeon, appears in the Surry County Records:
"This Indenture made the ffourth day of . . . in the yeare
of or Lord God 1657: Between Charles Clay of the one

---

[14]Northampton County Records, v. 1632-40, p. 144.
[15]Ibid., v. 1640-45, pp. 231-35; pp. 257-59.

ptie: & Stephen Tickner Chyrurgion of the other ptie:
Witnesseth That the sd Charles Clay doth hereby Covenant, grant & promise to & wth the sd Stephen Tickner, to
serve him or assigns in Such Imploymts as the sd Tickner
shall Employ him about in the way of Chyrurgerye, or
Phissicke, ffor & duringe the terme & time of seaven yeares
& the sd Tickner is to use his best skill & Judgmt to [teach]
him his Art, & what Cloathes the sd Charles doth bringe,
the sd Tickner is to returne to him at the Expiration of the
time afforesd. Signed: Charles Clay."[16]

There are few authentic instances of sons following their
fathers in the practice of medicine in these early years, but
such a development would be a natural outgrowth of the
apprentice system.   Probably more physicians than we know
followed the Hippocratic injunction, "I will impart a knowledge of the art to my own sons."   Dr. John Severne, who is
said to have received his medical education in Germany,
died in 1644, and his son is referred to in 1653 as "Dr.
John Severn."[17]

IV

Illiteracy was widespread in Virginia, as it was everywhere in this century.   On a coroner's jury in 1681 only
four out of twelve jurors could sign their names.   In the
same year only six out of eleven on a grand jury were able

---

[16]Surry County Records, v. 1, p. 109.
[17]Northampton County Records, v. 1640-45, pp. 275, 338.   Virginia
Magazine of History and Biography, v. 19, p. 105.

to write.[18]   In general about fifty percent of persons on juries could sign their names.   Of those making out deeds sixty percent of the men and thirty-three percent of the women were able to write.[19]   There were probably few physicians who found it necessary to make the familiar "His Mark."   We have discovered only one in the county records—Stephen Gill, who, although a Justice of York County in 1653 and a Burgess the same year, was apparently unable to sign his name.[20]   Sarah Overstreet, the wife of a physician, could not write.[21]   The usual indenture contract for children required the master to instruct them in the Ten Commandments and the Lord's Prayer, to teach them to read one chapter in the Bible, and to give them a new suit of clothes at the end of their period of servitude.   No stress, apparently, was put upon learning to write.

In spite of the rather widespread illiteracy the county records contain frequent references to books and libraries. Curious entries, usually found in wills and inventories, give us some insight into what must have been for many physicians their only theoretical training in medicine—the medical libraries of Seventeenth Century Virginians.

Of the libraries belonging to physicians none appears to have been large with the exception of Dr. Henry Willoughby's. In 1677 his estate included "44 books of Phisick," folio, quarto and octavo, valued at 631 pounds of

[18]Surry County Records, v. 2, p. 281.
[19]Bruce: Institutional History of Virginia, v. 1, p. 450.
[20]York County Records, v. 1, pp. 26, 28, 43, 55; v. 2, p. 88.
[21]Ibid., v. 5, p. 217.

tobacco; also seventy-four divinity books and thirty-eight law books.[22]   Many of the books mentioned in the inventories of doctors' estates were written in Latin or Dutch, and they are often referred to by the appraisers as being old and stored away in boxes.

Dr. Pott brought with him to the colony in 1621 medical books costing ten pounds, selected for him by Dr. Gulstone. Dr. John Holloway in 1643 left to John Tilney "all my phisicall and chirurgicall bookes Latin & English," thirteen volumes in all.[23]   Dr. John Severne left "1 parcell of old bookes" in 1644.[24]   Ralph Watson in 1645 left "thirty greate bookes in folio most of them . . . being Lattin bookes."[25]   In 1653 Stephen Gill, who could not sign his own name, left "one parcell of old books" worth 100 pounds of tobacco.[26]   Dr. Giles Modé had "Bookes in Dutch nothing English," valued at five shillings.[27]   Dr. Henry Waldron in 1657 bequeathed to Dr. Robert Ellyson "all my library of Bookes whatsoever in this country . . . together with my chests of physicall meanes. . . ."[28]   Dr. George Hacke left a large library, chiefly in German, in 1665.[29]   Dr. John Lee's library was valued at 4,000 pounds of tobacco in 1674.[30] Dr. Francis Haddon in 1680 left a "parcel of Latine

22Rappahannock County Records, v. 1677-82, p. 75.
23Northampton County Records, v. 1640-45, pp. 257-59.
24Northampton County Records, v. 1640-45, p. 338.
25York County Records, v. 2, p. 83.
26Ibid., v. 1, pp. 56-58.
27Ibid., v. 2, p. 58.
28Ibid., v. 3, p. 18.
29Bruce: Institutional History of Virginia, v. 1, p. 432.
30Ibid., p. 318.

books . . .," worth four pounds sterling.[31] James Love, ship surgeon, left by will "a large sedar chest full of Books, the catalogue of which books . . . is in a small chest."[32] Nathaniel Hill, school teacher and physician, had among other volumes "10 Physick books."[33] In 1691 Dr. Henry Power left a "Parcel of books," worth five pounds sterling.[34] Henry Andrews owned "7 large books in folio, 20 physick bks in Lattin, 45 small bookes."[35] Dr. Richard Starke left a "medson book."[36]

The inventories do not mention the titles of these books belonging to physicians, but in the library of the Richmond Academy of Medicine (Miller Collection) there are two medical books once owned by Seventeenth Century Virginia doctors. One is *A Description of the Body of Man,* by Helkiah Crooke, bearing on its title page the signature of Thomas Rootes, "Doc . . . in Physic," of Lancaster County, who died in 1660. The other is the works of Galen, which belonged to Thomas Robins, a York County chirurgeon who died in 1677.

Many citizens who were not doctors owned medical books whose titles have been preserved and which were probably similar to the books owned by physicians. There was a tendency toward self reliance in medical matters on the part of laymen, which became much more marked in the next

[31]York County Records, v. 5, p. 196.
[32]Rappahannock County Records, v. 7, p. 90.
[33]Henrico County Records, v. 5, p. 182.
[34]York County Records, v. 9, p. 293.
[35]William and Mary Quarterly, v. 2, p. 165.
[36]Virginia Magazine of History and Biography, v. 33, p. 27.

century. Well educated men like Richard Lee, who was an
Oxford graduate and a lifelong student, probably felt that
with the best English medical authorities on their shelves
they were safer than in the hands of the ignorant colonial
physician. William Byrd, the elder, had an aversion to
doctors which was inherited by his celebrated son. At the
time of his death he was alone at Westover with only his
housekeeper and his man. "He had been ill for some time,
being 'very lame of the gout' in 1700. . . . On Dec. 3, 1704
when he believed that death was upon him, he sent a boat
for Lieutenant William Randolph, who came at once . . .
To him Byrd gave some instructions as to his will and early
the next morning died."[37]   There is no record that he sent
for a doctor.

Among the lay Virginians whose libraries contained medical books were Matthew Hubbard, who owned five, and
John Kemp, who had "seven bookes of Chirurgerye."
Reverend Thomas Teackle had 100 volumes on medicine,
Colonel John Carter had five, Captain Thomas Carter two
or three, John Mottrom, William Fitzhugh and John Annis
each had one. Ralph Wormeley's library contained eighteen medical works, and Colonel Richard Lee's fourteen.
The titles of the various medical treatise, as given in the old
inventories, are interesting in spite of bad spelling:

Riverius's *Book of phisick*
    Lazarus Rivière (Riverius) in 1655 published a work

---

[37]Writings of Col. William Byrd of Westover, Introduction, p. xl.

on medicine which enjoyed the greatest popularity and which was translated into English by Culpeper in 1678.
Culpepps *Dispensatory,* folio
Culpeppers *Anatomy,* folio

Nicholas Culpeper in 1675 translated the *Pharmacopoeia Londinensis* into English. He was the "arch herbalist and quacksalver of the time, indulged in a vast amount of scurrilous raillery at the expense of the London Pharmacopœias of 1618 and 1650, but, except for his herb-lore, he was himself only the credulous astrologer described by Nedham, as a 'frowsy-headed coxcomb' who had 'gallimawfried the Apothecaries' Book into nonsense' in his aim to 'monopolize to himself all the knavery and cozenage that ever an apothecary's shop was capable of.' " (Garrison: History of Medicine, p. 291.)

Sennertus *Of the Scurvy*
Sennertus *Chirurgery*
Sennurtor *Institution of phisick*
Phisitians Library, folio
Doctr Willis *practice of Physick*

Thomas Willis, 1621-1675, leading exponent of chemistry, had the largest fashionable practice of London. His *Anatomy* gave the most complete and accurate account of the nervous system. He was a close clinical observer, like Sydenham. His *London Practice of Physic*, 1685, described *myasthenia gravis* for the first time. He was the first to notice the sweetish taste of diabetic urine.

Practice of Physick
Institution of Physick

An old Latin Physick Book
a Physick book
Dispenser
Naturall Magick
Ambrose Parry's *Chirurgery*
> Ambrose Paré, 1510-1590, French army barber-surgeon. Treated gunshot wounds without boiling oil, ligated blood vessels instead of cauterizing them, popularized podalic version, introduced new surgical instruments and methods. Author of an important work on surgery.

Pancraetick Juice
A treasis of the gout
The way to health long life and happiness
Byfield *upon Physick*
> Timothy Byfield's *sal oleosum volatile* was the first proprietary medicine patented in England to take advantage of the old statute of monopolies of 1624.

Gallons (Galen's) *art of Physick*
The unlearned Keymiss
The English Physician
Salmon's *Dispensatory*
> Peter Salmon, died 1675. M. D. from Padua, 1630. Fellow of College of Physicians. New London Dispensatory, 1678.

Poorman's Family Book
Boyle's *Letter to a Friend concerning Specific Physic*
Cooks *Anatomy*
> Helkiah Crooke, Scholar at St. John's, Cambridge, in 1591, M. D. 1604. In 1616 he wrote a *Description*

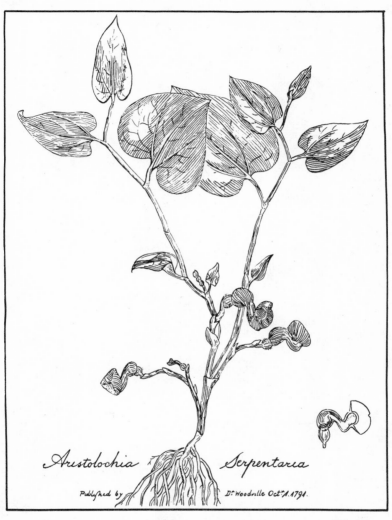

Aristolochia *Serpentaria*

Published by Dr Woodville Octr 1. 1791.

Snake Root, highly valued as a remedy in Seventeenth Century Virginia.

of the Body of Man, collected and translated out of all the best authors of anatomy.

French's *Art of Distillation*

Thoughts on Surgery

Surgeon Mate

John Woodall, 1556-1643, foremost 17th Century English Surgeon, wrote the *Surgeon's Mate,* which was published in 1617. In it is the earliest account of lemon juice in the treatment of scurvy.

Barrowes *Method of phisick*

Philip Barrow or Barrough, author of the *Method of Physick, contaning the Causes, Signes, and Cures of Inward Diseases in Man's Body from the head to the foote. Whereunto is added the forme and rule of making remedies and medicines, which our Physitions commonly use at this day, with the proportion, quantity, and names of each medicine,* published in London, 1590. It was dedicated to Lord Burghley, and reached its seventh edition in 1652. There are only two copies now in America.

Regimt of Health

The Regimen of Health was the output of the School of Salerno. There was an English translation in 1634.

Aristotles *problems*

Guielm Hardaei *Medici Regii*

Either William or Gideon Harvey.

Praxis Medicinae

A piece of Surgery

Exercitationes de morbis

Alberti Magni *opera*

Systema medicinale

Method of Physick

Bates *Dispensatory*

    William Bates, physician to Charles I and Charles II.

Glisson's *Anatomy*

    Francis Glisson, the foremost English anatomist.

Reconciliableness of Specifick Medicines

Corneli felsus *de Medicina*

    Cornelius Celsus.

Vigors *chirurgery*

    Juan de Vigo was influential in introducing cinchona bark into Europe. He was the most important surgeon from Guy de Chauliac to Paré, and was early interested in gunshot wounds and in syphilis. There were several translations and more than 200 editions of his *Surgery*, 1513-1600.

Of the Birth of Mankinde

    The *Rosengarten*, 1513, of Eucharius Rösslin was taken mainly from the remarkable treatise of Soranus of Ephesus (2nd Cent. A. D.). Thomas Raynold, 1545, translated Rösslin's work, and it was published in London under the title of *The Byrth of Mankynde*.

V

Looking back over the century we find that a few physicians undoubtedly held university degrees, but that the majority of them learned medicine in an apprenticeship either in England or in this country. There was in Virginia a well established free school system, where a preliminary education could be had, and physicians took an active part in these early schools. The system of indenture was common and trained many physicians, who during five to eight years of apprenticeship acquired what knowledge their masters possessed and then set up for themselves. There were no boards of examiners to detect and weed out the incompetent, and a man's declaration of his professional skill was the only license required.

That the medical training of the early colonial doctors was considered inadequate in their own day is shown by the remarks of two of their contemporaries. In 1683 acting-governor Nicholas Spenser, who was suffering from either disease of the gall bladder or nephritis, preferred long distance treatment from England to the ministrations of the local physicians, for he wrote to his brother: "I still remaine some what indisposed, and indeede doe dispaire of A remedy heere. I have heere stated unto you my distemper, concerning which please to advize with some able Physitian for mee.

"My chiefe griefe is the paine of the Hypocondriacke, with some tymes A swiming in my head and A paine in the hinder part of it, with often moderate paines occationed as I suppose by wind flyeing into my shoulders, backe and hipps; little Appety, and little sleepe, often A nautiateing of my victualls; very subiect to receive coulds and apt to be A little feaverish. My urin is Thin, and pale. In A morning when I first rise I am apt to be troubled with A trembleing in my limbs. By what I can understand of my distempers it proceeds from obstructions of spleen, Liver and Messeraicke veines. . . ."[38]

Early in the next century we find William Byrd II writing to Sir Hans Sloane: "Here be some men indeed that are call'd Doctors: but they are generally discarded Surgeons of Ships, that know nothing above very common Remedys. They are not acquainted enough with Plants or other parts of Natural History, to do any Service to the World, which makes me wish that we had some missionary Philosopher, that might instruct us in the many usefull things which we now possess to no purpose."[39]

---

[38]William and Mary Quarterly, second series, v. 3, p. 135.
[39]Ibid., second series, v. 1, pp. 186-191.

CHAPTER IV

SIMPLES AND THERAPY

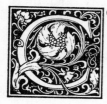ONTROL of the trade routes and drug marts of the world passed into the hands of the Dutch and the English in the Seventeenth Century.[1] Portugal, Spain, England and Holland had each attempted to circumvent the Venetian trade through Egypt with India by discovering some new and more direct route. Commercial rivalry was keen. Spices and drugs as well as gold and precious stones lured on the explorer. The English were the last to sense the importance of this trade. At first they were content to capture Dutch and Portuguese vessels laden with these precious objects. But with a colony on the shores of Virginia they soon appreciated the possibilities of developing a drug trade of their own and of discovering new and potent herbs. That the rivalry with other countries continued into the Eighteenth Century is shown in a letter from Sir Hans Sloane to William Byrd II in 1709: "I have heard that the Dutch have been at Immense expences in destroying the Spice trees in the E. Indies and that yet they cannot lessen their annuall expences upon that acct. I mentn. these particulars that you may look abt & I dare say you will find plenty of it [Ipecoacanna, which could be sold at thirty shillings a pound] & you will save so

---

[1]Garrison: History of Medicine, p. 294.

much money as goes from hence to Prtugall & Spain on this Occasion."[2]

Thomas Harriot, who describes himself as "seruant to Sir Walter Raleigh, a member of the Colony, and there employed in discovering," is enthusiastic in his descriptions of minerals and drugs encountered in the new country.[3] He describes the virtues of rock alum, plain alum,[4] a kind of clay called *wapeib* which the inhabitants used "for the cure of sores and woundes," sassafras,[5] which he considers better than guaiacum, and sweet gums and tobacco.

Whitaker's *Good News from Virginia* in 1612 says: "What should I name unto you the divers sorts of trees, sweete woods and Physicall plants: the divers kind of Oakes and Walnut trees. The Pines, Pitch-Trees, Soape-ashes trees, Sassafras, Cedar, Ash, Maple, Cypress, and many more. . . ."[6]

Hartwell, Chilton and Blair, writing much later, declare

---

[2]William and Mary Quarterly, second series, v. 1, p. 191.

[3]Harriot: A Briefe and True Report of the New Found Land of Virginia, 1586.

[4]Ibid., p. 15. "There is a veine of earth along the sea coast for the space of fourtie or fiftie miles, whereof by the judgement of some that haue made triall heere in England is made good *Allum*, of the kind which is called *Roche Allum*. The richnesse of such a commoditie is so well knowne that I neede not saye anything thereof. The same earth doth also yealde *White Copresse, Nitrum,* and *Alumen plumeum,* but nothing so plentifully as the common *Allum;* which be also of price and profitable."

[5]Ibid., p. 16. "Called by the inhabitants *Winauk,* a kinde of wood of most pleasant and sweete smel; and of most rare vertues in phisick for the cure of many diseases. It is foud by experience to bee farre better and of more uses then the wood which is called *Guaiacum* or *Lignum vitae.*"

[6]Brown: Genesis of the U. S., v. 2, p. 587.

"it is an excellent country for dyeing stuff and curious simples."

In June 1613 Sir Samuel Argoll writes of his voyage to Virginia: "In this Journie I likewise found . . . a strange kind of Earth, the vertue whereof I know not; but the Indians eate it for Physicke, alleaging that it cureth the sicknesse and paine of the belly. I likewise found a kind of water issuing out of the Earth, which hath a tart taste much like unto Allum-water, it is good and wholesome: for my men did drinke much of it, and never found it otherwise. I also found an earth like a Gumme, white and cleere; another sort of red like Terra sigillata; another very white, and of so light a substance, that being cast into the water, it swimmeth."[7]

Such glowing accounts as these stirred the London Company to action, and in 1619 instructions were forwarded to Virginia advising the colony what plants were considered valuable and how they should be prepared for shipping: "1. Small sassafras rootes to be drawen in the winter and dryed and none to be medled with in the Sommer, and it is worthe 50 lb. and better per Tonne. 3. Poccone to be gotten from the Indians and put up in caske is worthe per Tonne 11 lb. 4. Galbrand groweth like fennell in fashion, and there is greatest stoare of it in Warriscoes Country, where they cut walnut trees laste. You must cut it downe in Maye or June, and beinge downe it is to be cut into small

---

[7]Brown: Genesis of the U. S., v. 2, p. 642.

peeces, and brused and pressed in your small presses, the juice thereof is to be saved and put into casks, which wilbe worthe here per Tonne, 100 lb. at leaste. 5. Sarsapilla is a Roote that runneth within the grounds like unto Licoras, which beareth a small rounde leafe close by the grounde, which being founde the Roote is to be pulled up and dryed and bounde up in bundles like faggotts, this is to be done towards the ende of Sommer before the leafe fall from the stalk; and it is worthe here per Tonne, 200 lb. 6. Wallnutt oyle is worth here 30 lb. per Tonne, and the like is chestnutt oyle and chechinkamyne oyle."[8]

The London Company in 1621 sent out Sir Francis Wyatt with orders to search the country for minerals, drugs, gums and the like. As a result we find Governor Wyatt in 1622 issuing this order to ensign John Uty at Hogg Island: "Whereas we have received commaund from the right honourable the Earle of Southampton for the sending home of threescore thousand waight of Sasafras: These are . . . therfore to charge and commaund you Mr. Uty, that for every fiveteene you leavy one thousand waight of good Sasafrax, viz, for every man 66 pounds waight a piece, which must be brought aboard the Abigail, before the first day of March next, on paine of every hundreth waight so wanting, to forfeit ten pounds of Tobacco. The size of the Sasafrax must not exceede the bignes of a mans arme. Given at James Citty this 14th of February Anno Domini 1622. . ."[9]

8Brown: Genesis of the U. S., v. 1, p. 384.
9William and Mary Quarterly, second series, v. 8, pp. 51, 54, 55.

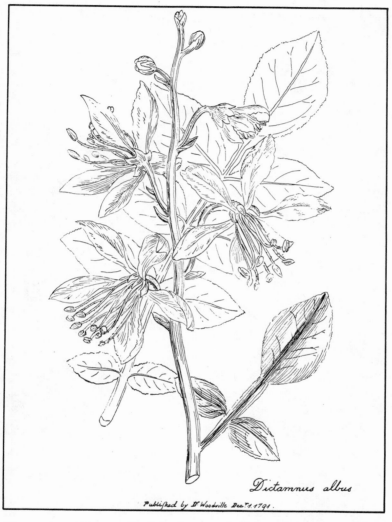

Dictamnus albus

Published by D.ʳ Woodville Dec.ᵗ 1. 1791.

Dittany, frequently prescribed by Seventeenth Century Virginia physicians.

A year later Governor Wyatt is still trying to collect fines from those who have not brought in their sixty-six pounds of sassafras.

A letter from the Company to the colonial authorities, July 25, 1621, prays "you all in generall that such extraordinary oare or earth as you find you send us over in plentie, for that which was sent by your Capt. Nuce was in so small proportion as we hardly could make any triall thereof; we conceive it to be Terra Lemnia and it is exceeding good for the flux, youe shall therefore do well to bring it into use in the Colony: we desire youe Captain Newce therefore to send us over three or foure Tunne of the said white earth. . . ."[10]

In 1621 it was urged in an article on Virginia that no contemptible profit "may be made of Woods, if by boaring holes in divers trees, of whose vertues wee are yet ignorant, and collecting the juce thereof, a scrutiny be made which are fit for Medicinall liquor and Balsomes; which for gummes, Perfumes, and Dyes, and heere I may justly take occasion to complain of our owne sloth and indulgence, if compared to the laborious Spanyard, who by this very practice have found out many excellent Druggs, Paints and Colours meerely by bruizing and grinding Woods. . . . The French relations of their Voyages to Canada, tell us that the Indians and themselves falling into a contagious disease, of which Phisitians could give no Reason or Remedy, they were all in a short

---

[10]Neill: Virginia Company of London, p. 228.

space restored to their health meerly by drinking water, in which Saxifrage was infused and boyled, which was then discovered to them by the Natives, and wee justly entertaine beliefe that many excellent Medicines either for conservation of Nature in her vigour or restauration in her decadence may be communicated unto us, if projection of this stampe be so much incouraged by hopes or reward of honour, as to be put in practice."[11]

In an appeal to the colonists in 1621 to send home specimens of the native simples the Company furnished "a valuation of the Commodities growing and to be had in Virginia." Mastic was said to bring three shillings a pound, wild sarsaparilla five shillings a hundred, domestic sarsaparilla ten shillings a hundred, while "red earth allenagra" brought three shillings a hundred. Red alum, called "carthagena allum," and "roach" alum, called "Romish allum," brought ten shillings the hundred. The colonists were directed to send sweet gums, roots, woods and berries for dyes and drugs, "all sorts as much as you can, every sort by it selfe, there being great quantities of those things in Virginia, which after proof made, may be heere valued to their worth. And particularly, we have great hope of the Pocoon root, that it will prove better than Madder."[12]

This interest in the drug possibilities of the colony continues throughout the century. There is a letter in 1660 from a certain Mr. Povey, written on behalf of the Royal

---

[11]Force: Tracts, v. 3, "Virginia Richly and Truly Valued," p. 15.
[12]Ibid., pp. 51, 52.

Society, inquiring into the natural products of Virginia and explaining that His Majesty, Charles II, "hath ordered a Garden purposely for Plants, and Simples, and varieties of that nature; and it will bee most acceptable to his Ma'tie if any thing of that kind may bee presented to him from Virginia." Enclosed with the letter were some "enquiryes concerning those severall kind of things which are reported to be in Virginia & the Bermudas, not found in England:"

"1. Concerning the variety of earths. 'Tis said there is one kinde of a Gummy consistence, white & cleere another white & so light that it swims uppon water, another red called Wapergh like terra Sigillita."

"2. What considerable mineralls, stones, Bitumens, tinctures, Drugges, & a specimen of each.
What hot Bathes, & of what medicinall use."

"3. What variety of Plants are native there & not in England, what kind of peculiar herbs there are, considerable either for their flower, smell, Alimentary or medicinall use." "So tis said that in the Bermudas there is a poison weede like our Ivy whose leaves doe by the touch cause blisters. A red reed whose juice or infusion causeth vomit. A kind of woodbine, whose fruite like a flat beane, purgeth vehemently."

"What kind of animalls. . . . Insects, flyes, ants, wormes, Spiders. Some of each kind to be sent over either alive or dead."

"Whether Deere have generally 3 or 4 fawnes at a broode, & whether any of the Cattle transported from hence, become there more fruitfull than they were here."

"Whether the Dogs barke not, but only howle as wolves."
"Whether the Natives be borne White."[13]

In 1668 Dr. Benjamin Worseley was granted a monopoly in the cultivation of senna in the colony: "Warrant to the Attorney or Solicitor General. To prepare a bill containing his Majesty's grant of special license to Benjamin Worseley, Doctor of Physic, and his assigns, for the sole use of his invention of planting, dressing, and curing Senna in his Majesty's Plantations in America for 14 years, with a prohibition to all others within his Majesty's dominions during said term without license of said Dr. Worseley or his assigns."[14]

An item in a letter from Captain William Byrd of Westover to Thomas Gower in England, May 20, 1684, shows that the search for native simples had enlisted the cooperation of prominent Virginians. "I designed you a Parcell of Snake-root," he writes, "but Wynne hurrying his boat away, it is left behind; hee pretends his ship is so full hee cannot carry it."[15]

The *Philosophical Transactions* of the Royal Society for 1690 contain the following articles which prove the interest of Englishmen in the botany and biology of the new world:

"The Method the Indians in Virginia and Carolina use to Dress Buck and Doe-Skins; as it was communicated to the

---

[13]William and Mary Quarterly, second series, v. 1, p. 66.
[14]Calendar British State Papers, America and West Indies, v. 1661-68, p. 604.
[15]Virginia Historical Register, v. 1, p. 114.

Royal Society by the Honourable Sir Robert Southwell, Knt. their President."

"Some Experiments on a Black Shining Sand brought from Virginia, supposed to contain Iron, made in March 1689. By Allen Moulen, M. D. and Fellow of the Royal Society, since dead." (The experiments unfortunately gave negative results.)

"The Description of the American Tomineius, or Humming Bird, communicated by Nehemiah Grew, M. D. and Fellow of the Royal Society."[16]

The search for new things in Virginia led to experiments of various sorts. Among these were the distillation projects of Mr. Russell. In July 1620 this "acmunist and chemist" proposed to John Smith of Nibley to supply the colony with an artificial wine, to be made in Virginia from a vegetable which grew there. It could be made cheaply and easily, would keep well, and would not intoxicate. Russell asked a thousand pounds for it of the Company; but on April 12, 1621, Sir John Brooke told Smith that "of his own knowledge this wine was made of Sassaphras, & Licoras boyled in water; he had of the drink."[17]

In December 1620 Captain George Thorpe wrote to England that he was "persuaded that more do die here of the disease of their minds than of their body . . . and by not knowing they shall [have to] drink water here." When "Mr. Russell the chimist" was trying to introduce sassafras

---

[16]Philosophical Transactions, 1690, v. 17, 18.
[17]Brown: First Republic, p. 395.

tea into Virginia as an artificial wine in July 1620, it was stated that "there is in Virginia and is like to be shortly 3,000 people. And the greatest want they complayne of is good drinke, wine beinge too dear, and barley chargeable, which though it should there be sowen, it were hard in that Country, being so hot, to make malt of it, or if they had malt to make good beer." But, Thorpe added, "they had found a way to make a good drink from Indian corn, which he prefered to good English beer." This may have been the beginning of old Virginia corn whiskey, for this use of corn had long been known. Goncalo Ximines, of New Granada, who died in 1546, wrote that "maize steeped in water, boiled, and afterwards fermented makes a very strong liquor."[18]

Out of this search for health-giving and health-restoring plants and minerals very little of permanent value resulted, though the virtues of snake-root, dittany, turbith and mechoacon, fever and ague root, senna, lemnian earth, alum, sweet gums and tobacco continued to be extolled and enthusiastically advocated.

Among the simples popular in the colony one of the earliest discovered and sent home in great quantities was sassafras. The first letter ever written by the Council to the Company describes how demoralizing was the finding of such an abundant quantity in this country: ". . . our easiest and richest commodity being Sasafrix roots were gathered

---

[18]Brown: First Republic, p. 409.

up by the Sailors with loss and spoil of our tools and with drawing of our men from our labor. We wish that they may be dealt with so that all the loss neither fall on us nor them. I believe they have thereof two tunnes at least which if they scatter abroad at their pleasure will pull down our price for a long time, we leave this to your wisdomes."[19] The pith, when mixed with water, formed a mucilage which was used in diseases of the eye and as a drink in dysentery and nephritis. The bark, which was sweet, fragrant and aromatic, was employed as a stimulant and astringent. Sassafras was said to be useful in skin diseases, gout, rheumatism and syphilis. At one time it was commonly sold at daybreak in London under the name of Saloop, and until fairly recently saloop venders were found there.

Snake root, *serpentaria,* was said to have a tonic, diuretic, diaphoretic and stimulant effect and was popular in typhoid and digestive disorders. Black snake root, *radex serpentaria nigra,* was a remedy for gout, rheumatism and amenorrhoea. Mr. Thomas Glover, who is described as "an ingenious chirurgeon that hath lived some years in that country," sent an account of Virginia to the Royal Society in 1676. He notes that "here groweth the Radex Serpentaria Nigra, which was so much used in the last great pestilence, that the price of it advanced from ten shillings to three pounds sterling a pound."[20] Beverley years later wrote, "There is the snake root so much admired in Eng-

---

[19]Stanard: Virginia's First Century, p. 40.
[20]Glover: Account of Virginia, p. 17.

land as a cordial and being a great antidote in all pestilent disorders," and "there's the rattlesnake root, to which no remedy was ever yet found comparable; for it effectually cures the bite of a rattlesnake which sometimes has been mortal in two minutes. If this medicine be early applied, it presently removes the infection, and in two or three hours restores the patient to as perfect health as if he had never been hurt."[21]

Thomas Glover describes four other popular simples—dittany, turbith, mechoacon, and the fever and ague root. "Here is also an herb which some call Dittany, others Pepper-wort; it is not Dittany of Candia, nor English Dittander; it groweth a foot or a foot and a half high, the leaves are about the bredth of a groat, and figur'd like a heart, and short out of the stalk and branches one of a side directly opposite each other, it smelleth hot like pepper and biteth upon the Tongue. The water of this herb distill'd out of a Limbeck, is one of the best things I know of to drive worms out of the Body; and an ounce of this water taken, provoketh sweat plentifully. Here grow two Roots which some physicians judg, the one to be Turbith, the other Mechoacon, but they be right or no, I could not well judg. Both these Roots are purging and in their operations much like those we have at the Apothecaries, only somewhat more forcible, the reason may be because we have them more new and succulent. Here groweth a plant about a

---

[21]Beverley: History of Virginia, pp. 109, 110.

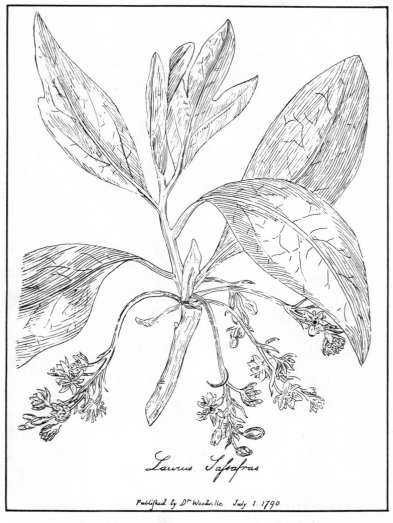

Laurus Sassafras

Published by Dr Woodville   July 1. 1790

Sassafras, which enjoyed a unique reputation as a medicine in
Seventeenth Century Virginia.

foot and a half or two foot in height, the leaves are rugg'd
like to a Borage leaf, but they are longer, and not above two
fingers broad; about the stalks, where the leaves grow out,
there hang berries, which being ripe are yellow. The English call it the Fever and Ague-root. This root being newly
taken out of the ground, and a dram and half of it infused
in beer or water the space of twelve hours, purgeth down-
ward with some violence, but I have given a dram of the
Root in powder, and then it only moveth sweat, and that
but moderately. It is a little bitter in taste and therefore
somewhat hot."[22]

Harriot lauds the healthful qualities of tobacco, "which
purgeth superfluous fleame & other grosse humors, openeth
all the pores & passages of the body: by which meanes
the use thereof, not only preserveth the body from obstructions; but also if any be, so that they have not beene
of too long continuance, in short time breaketh them:
whereby their bodies are notably preserved in health, and
know not many greevous diseases wherewithall wee in England are oftentimes afflicted."[23] Smokers swore it was
an "antidote to all poisons; that it expelled rheums, sour
humours, and obstruction of all kinds, and healed wounds
better than St. John's wort. Some doctors were of opinion
it would heal gout and the ague, neutralize the effects of
drunkeness and remove weariness and hunger." In England
the apothecaries sold the best tobacco and became masters

---

[22]Glover: Account of Virginia, pp. 17, 18.
[23]Harriot: Briefe and True Report, etc., p. 30.

of the art of smoking. They received pupils, whom they taught to exhale the smoke in little globes, rings or the "Euripus." These tricks were called "the slights."[24]

The Jamestown weed, called *datura stramonium,* is at first sedative and antispasmodic, in larger doses a narcotic and poisonous. Beverley's account of its effect on certain soldiers is undoubtedly overdrawn: "The Jamestown weed (which resembles the thorny apple of Peru, and I take to be the plant so called) is supposed to be one of the greatest coolers in the world. This being an early plant, was gathered very young for a boiled salad by some of the soldiers sent thither to quell the rebellion of Bacon; and some of them eat plentifully of it, the effect of which was a very pleasant comedy; for they turned natural fools upon it for several days: one would blow up a feather in the air; another would dart straws at it with much fury; and another stark naked was sitting up in a corner, like a monkey, grinning and making mows at them; a fourth would fondly kiss and paw his companions, and snear in their faces, with a countenance more antic than any in a Dutch droll. In this frantic condition they were confined, lest they should in their folly destroy themselves; though it was observed that all their actions were full of innocence and good nature. Indeed, they were not very cleanly, for they would have wallowed in their own excrements if they had not been prevented. A thousand such simple tricks they played, and

---

[24]Virginia Magazine of History and Biography, v. 29, p. 107.

after eleven days returned to themselves again, not remembering anything that had passed."[25]

Beverley also extols the wild cherry bark as a substitute for *cortex peruviana* and the powdered bark of the prickly ash as a specific in "old wounds and long running sores."

We naturally search the records for other familiar drugs, some of which were just coming into notice, others having been known from the earliest times. Ipecac, a medicine much prized by Colonel Byrd in the next century, was a secret remedy for dysentery until 1688, when the French Government paid 20,000 francs for it. Antimony, though it enjoyed a great vogue during the century and was famous at the French Court, is not mentioned in the Virginia records. Cinchona bark was introduced into England about the middle of the Seventeenth Century. It was denounced there by many physicians because it was supposed to "fix the humour." Sydenham in 1668 declared that "some had been killed by having it given just before the fit." It was 1676 before the first English physician of his day came out squarely in favor of it. It is easy to understand, therefore, why there are no references to cinchona bark in Seventeenth Century Virginia. It was probably very late in the century before it was used in this country.

Castor oil is not mentioned, though it had been known since the time of Egyptian medicine. There is no indication of what the Virginia "purge" was, but colycinth had been

---

[25]Beverley: History of Virginia, p. 110.

prescribed since the days of Rufus of Ephesus. Aloes was a product of the Barbadoes, and senna was actively cultivated in the colony. Rhubarb is frequently mentioned. Cascara is not referred to.

Among the stimulants caffeine was not known, because tea and coffee had probably not been introduced. Nux vomica was native in India and China, and is not mentioned. Aromatic spirits of ammonia was not familiar to the Virginia doctor, as Clayton emphatically asserts. They did know the use of spirits and opium, and of at least one of the belladonna group, Jamestown weed. Alum, which was common, must have been an important element in the astringent preparations so frequently prescribed. Whether the tonics given contained iron, which Sydenham was vigorously advocating during this century, is not known. There is no mention of calomel, the Sampson of the medicine of the next century, though it had long before been recommended by Paracelsus. Of course there was no digitalis, no antiseptics, no glandular products, no anaesthetics, no coal tar products, none of that great group of synthetic medicines which still knock daily at the door of the modern pharmacopeia.

The Reverend John Clayton has left an illuminating account of the elaborate methods of treatment he himself used, particularly in the matter of dogbites. For hydrophobia he prescribed the volatile salts of amber, ten grains in treacle water every half hour. To this was added "posset drink" (sour milk) with sage and rue. Clayton said that a doctress of his acquaintance treated snake bite with "Oriental Bezoar shaved and a decoction of dittany." He recommends chalybeates, decoctions, carminative seeds and aromatic spirits. "But," he says, "their [Virginia] Doctors are so learned, that I never met with any of them that understood what Armoniack Spirits were: Two or three of them one time ran me clear down by Consent, that they were Vomitive, and that they never used any thing for that Purpose but Crocus Metallorum, which indeed every House keeps; and if their Finger, as the Saying is, ake but, they immediately give three or four Spoonfuls thereof; if this fail, they give him a second Dose, then perhaps Purge them with fifteen or twenty Grains of the Rosin of Jalap, afterwards Sweat them with Venice treacle, Powder of Snakeroot, or Gascoin's Powder; and when these fail conclamatum est."[26]

Gascoin's powder must have been one of those proprietary preparations so common in a century famous for its nostrums. There were Scot's Pills and Daffy's Elixir, Dutch Drops, Goddard's Drops, Seignette's Salts and a host of others. On the whole, however, the therapeutics of the Virginia physician were simple. The weighty hand of Arabian polypharmacy, as Osler called it, does not appear to have rested very heavily upon them. There were two reasons for this. Drugs were very expensive, especially those which had to be imported, and apothecaries were scarce, particularly toward the end of the century. Most of the medicines given

---

[26]Clayton: Letter to the Royal Society, 1688; in Force: Tracts, v. 3, p. 6.

by Virginia doctors were extremely plain and were com-
pounded at home.

In the earliest years of the century there were several
apothecaries in the colony. Thomas Field and Thomas
Harford came over with the first settlers, and Fitch and
Townshend were apothecaries to John Pott. But by 1621
there was a great scarcity, as the following will show: "It
was signified unto the Court that an Apothecary offered to
transport himself and his wife at his own charge to Virginia
if the Company would please to give them their transport of
two children, the one being under the age of eight and the
other a youth of good years: which offer the Court did very
well like of in respect of the great want of men of his profession, and being put to the question did agree thereunto;
provided that the Apothecary at his coming over did exercise his skill and practise in that profession. . . ."[27]

There is no further record of apothecaries living in the
colony in this century. John Hubbard of York County, who
in 1688 left "2 boxes of phisicke," valued at 15 lb. sterling,
was probably a merchant. It later became common practice
in Virginia for grocers to import drugs for sale to doctors
and the public. Grocers were the original apothecaries and
were first incorporated in England in 1345. The Seventeenth Century Virginia physician was for the most part his
own apothecary. The medical equipment listed in inventories of Virginia physicians includes such items as "one

---

[27]Records of the Virginia Company, v. 1, p. 495.

small brasse mortar & pestle on pewter," owned by George Hopkins in 1644;[28] "a small box with some phisick salves, old scales & a salvatory bottles & a gallipots," Matthew Hubbard, 1667;[29] "one small brass mortar and pestle . . . one cesterne . . . gallipots and glasses," John Holloway;[30] "1 pr brass scales . . . one pr gold weights," John Severne, 1644;[31] "a box of small violls," Henry Willoughby, 1685;[32] "An old phisick chest with empty pot and glass of several compositions medicines & utensils thereto appertayning . . .," Andrew Winter, 1679;[33] "Old phisick chest with drugs in it . . . small box with phisic," Stephen Gill, 1653;[34] "A large Bell Mettall mortar," Richard Starke;[35] "And one box of medicines and 2 searses and 2 old cases with bottles and one barbers empty case," George Gunnell.[36]

With this equipment we find Virginia physicians prescribing purges, cordial and astringent boluses, opiate and purging pills, juleps,[37] cordial waters, confections and spirits; also vomiting, purging, cordial[38] and cephalick[39] electuaries;[40] pectoral[41] and laxative syrups; cephalick, astringent,

[28]York County Records, v. 2, p. 85.
[29]Ibid., v. 4., p. 464.
[30]Northampton County Records, v. 1640-45, pp. 285, 287.
[31]Ibid., p. 338.
[32]Rappahannock County Records, v. 1677-82, p. 75.
[33]York, v. 6, p. 171.
[34]Ibid., v. 1, pp. 56-58.
[35]Ibid., v. 12, p. 317.
[36]Elizabeth City County Records, v. 1684-99, p. 294.
[37]Julep—a sweet drink.
[38]Cordial—tonic.
[39]Cephalick—for headache.
[40]Electuary—a confection.
[41]Pectoral—pertaining to affections of the chest.

stomatic and cordial powders; oxymel,[42] ursicatories, defensives,[43] ointments, oiles and external applications.

George Wale in York County prescribed "torrefyed rubub, opiate pills, opiate cordial, potions with rhubarb and mirab, electuaries, and astringent boles."[44] John Clulo's therapy consisted of "stringent potions, cordial Astringent boles, cordyall Iulebs."[45] Patrick Napier was fond of giving various cordials, "pectoral meanes" and the celebrated electuary, Confectio Alkermes.[46] Daniel Parke used cordial waters, spirits of cinnamon, cordial boles, oils and spirits.[47] Jeremiah Rawlins prescribed cordials, boles, "a purge of Rhubarb & Morabalans."[48] Giles Modé dispensed electuaries for vomiting, juleps, laxatives, syrups and stomach powders.[49] Jeoffrey Wilson comforted a patient with a narcotic cordial in addition to "Barley att times for drinke, mace, nuttmegs, licorice, Oyle of Roses & Camon."[50] Francis Haddon, in addition to cordials, purges and electuaries, used ointments, defensives, cephalick and astringent powders and other "Externall Applications."[51] In a day of almost pure symptomatic therapy the colonial doctor evidently had considerable range and variety in his treatment of disease.

---

[42]Honey and vinegar boiled to a syrupy consistency.
[43]Agents used over wounds to keep out air.
[44]York County Records, v. 3, p. 67.
[45]Ibid., v. 3, p. 66.
[46]Ibid., v. 4, p. 169.
[47]Ibid., v. 3, p. 220.
[48]Ibid., v. 3, p. 259.
[49]Ibid., v. 2, p. 69.
[50]Ibid., v. 3, p. 90.
[51]Ibid., v. 4, p. 442.

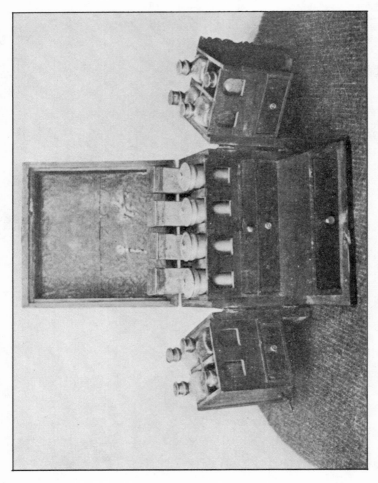

(*Library of the Richmond Academy of Medicine, Miller Collection.*)

Seventeenth Century medicine chest, open.

CHAPTER V

MEDICAL PRACTICE

I

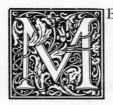EDICINE, like the other arts and sciences, emerged from the Middle Ages blighted by centuries of mental inertia. The rise of the universities, printing, the new learning and exploration helped to strike fire into a lethargic world. Before medicine could avail herself of the new freedom she had to reckon with a vast substratum of superstition and pedantry. The world was thronging with quacks. The heavy hand of monastic authority and the fetters of tradition forged more than a thousand years before were still felt.

The century before 1600 saw the new spirit at work in medicine. In spite of many surviving evils—alchemy, astrology, neo-platonism, witches, martyrs, dissolute itinerant medical students, peripatetic professors, uroscopy and herb doctors—we are indebted to the period for at least three signal contributions. These were the overthrow of authority, accurate anatomical descriptions based on human dissection, and the birth of surgery as a specialty of dignity and value. Paracelsus (1493-1541) in spite of his near-quackery was a rare and forceful personality, with a native medical instinct and full of the spirit of revolt. He succeeded in smashing the stupefying reverence for authority and popularized chemical studies of vast importance in medicine. The therapeutics of the next century is indebted to him for sulphur, mercury, calomel, zinc, laudanum, iron, antimony, arsenic, copper and the tinctures. The Sixteenth Century produced a greater man in Vesalius (1513-1564). With him accurate knowledge of the body structure was for the first time presented and the errors of Galen, which had passed unchallenged for a thousand years, were courageously exposed. With Fabricius, Fallopius, Eustachius, Sylvius and others the foundation of modern anatomy was laid. Finally, Ambrose Paré (1510-1590) made suffering humanity eternally grateful to him for his epoch-making contributions in popularizing podalic version, substituting soothing applications for boiling oil in the treatment of gunshot wounds, and using the ligature rather than the cautery in the treatment of hemorrhage after amputation.

We come upon Seventeenth Century medicine with expectations of further progress. It was the century of Harvey and the discovery of the circulation of the blood, and of the rise of the new physiology. In this century the microscope was perfected and the first bacteria seen. With the microscope came histology, and the father of this science was one of the ornaments of Seventeenth Century medicine. Marcello Malphighi's (1628-1694) studies of the chick embryo, the skin, the red blood cells, the taste buds of the tongue, the finer structures of the lungs, kidney and liver, as well as the demonstration of the capillaries were all made before 1700. In this same century lived Thomas Sydenham (1624-1689), the English Hippocrates, whose wholesome influence lingers today in his stress on the value of observation, bedside notes and the expectant treatment. To him we owe the modern management of tuberculosis, the recognition of scarlet fever, the use of iron in anemia, and the whole science of epidemiology.

Anatomy, which had made such strides in the preceding century, now claimed Glisson, Steno, Ruysch, Vieussens, Schneider, Peyer, Brunner, Wharton, Highmore, Redi, de Graaf, Swammerdam, Aselli, Pecquet, Wirsung, Bartholin, Nuck, Cowper, Bidloo, Meibom, Willis and others, a roll call of anatomical immortals.

Chemistry, which Paracelsus had set on its feet, became a real science in the Seventeenth Century. Rudolph Glauber (1604-1688) discovered the cathartic properties of sodium sulphate (Glauber's Salts). Van Helmont (1577-1644) was the discoverer of CO_2 and coined the word "gas." But many, including van Helmont and the fashionable London physician, Thomas Willis, attempted to apply the chemical theory to all disease. The results were fantastic, and their so-called *Iatrochemical* school added another incubus to medical progress. Similar extremes followed in the wake of physics. Boyle, Hooke and Sanctorius each made contributions, out of enthusiasm for which arose the *Iatrophysical* school with the doctrine that the laws of physics could be rigidly applied to all physiological phenomena. The theory reached ridiculous extremes in the teachings of

George Baglivi (1688-1706), which represented the vascular system as a hydraulic machine, the respiratory system as a balloon and the digestive system as a sieve. Every age has had its schools. *Methodism, Empiricism, Pneumatism, Solidism, Humoralism, Ecclecticism* cluttered medical progress during the first centuries of the Christian era. What *Brunonianism* was in the Eighteenth Century and *Hahnemannism* in the Nineteenth the *Iatrophysical* and *Iatrochemical* schools were in the Seventeenth Century.

Physiology was advanced by the work of Descartes and Bohn. Harvey made a valuable contribution on animal generation. Lower successfully attempted the first transfusion, and Sir Christopher Wren the first intravenous medication. Mayow all but discovered pulmonary oxidation. Harris, one of the earliest of the pediatricians, lived and wrote about children. The belief in spontaneous generation continued until the time of Pasteur, but in this century Francesco Redi launched an attack on the fallacious doctrine. Superstition was still rampant, belief in alchemy, magic and judicial astrology was common. The King's Evil and the popular faith in the royal touch reached their climax.

The Pharmacopeia of the century was enriched by the addition of Glauber's Salts, 1658, cinchona bark, 1632, ipecac, 1672, and tartar emetic, 1631. Antimony had a tremendous vogue. Digitalis was as yet unknown. The first London pharmacopeia was issued in 1618, another edition in 1650 and a third in 1675. Other English medical books of the century were Harvey's *De Motu Cordis,* 1628, and his *De Generatione Animalium*, 1651; Bidloo's *Anatomia*, 1685; Cowper's *Anatomy of Human Bodies*, 1698; Hooke's *Micrographia*, 1665; Thomas Willis's *London Practice of Physic*, 1685; Platter's *Praxis Medicae*, 1602-08; Salmon's *London Dispensatory*, 1678; James Yonge's *Triumphal Chariot of Turpentine*, 1679; Stephen Bradwell's *Helps in Suddain Accidents*, 1633; and Sydenham's *Opera Universa*, 1685. Some of these works were to be found in Seventeenth Century Virginia libraries.

A striking characteristic of medicine on the Continent in this century was the distinction which was everywhere made between the physician, the surgeon and the barber. This was particularly true in France. Here an aristocracy of physicians held aloof from the despised surgeons and barbers, and the surgeons in turn looked disdainfully on the humbler barbers. In England the barbers and surgeons were united by law into the Company of Barber Surgeons, but the union was distasteful to the surgeons and was dissolved in 1740. The inferior status of both callings is defined by Garrison when he says that "the general run of surgeons was still roughly classed with the horde of barbers, bath-keepers, executioners, and vagrant mountebanks" and "the surgeon was still under the ban unless needed in war time."

Besides their surgeons the English colonists brought to Virginia one barber, showing that even in this new settlement they were to recognize the distinction; but we hear little of barbers after their landing. The term "barber surgeon" does not seem to have been used in the colonial records. The surgeon was called "chirurgeon," a word derived from two Greek roots meaning respectively "hand" and "work." He was thought of as a hand worker, and his art as a kind of handicraft. A distinction was made in the colony between him and the more esteemed physician, who was called "doctor." The two titles frequently occur in the records, although Toner states that the title of doctor was not used in the colonies until 1769.[1] This statement, though quoted by other American medical historians, is undoubtedly an error, for a tabulation of the titles in the Virginia county records shows the title of doctor used as often as that of chirurgeon. Consistency in the use of the terms is often lacking, a man referred to as a chirurgeon in one portion of the record being called doctor in another. It is clear, however, that there was a difference in their standing, and as evidence of the superior value attached to the physician's service we have the Virginia fee bill of 1736, which allowed those practitioners who had had university training to charge twice the fee of those who had not.[2]

II

In a fascinating study in paleopathology Elliot Smith has shown on Egyptian mummies that these ancient people suffered and died from modern diseases such as arterio sclerosis

---

[1] Baas: Outlines of the History of Medicine and the Medical Profession.
[2] Walsh says that in New York barbers were confused with surgeons and were therefore called upon by the ignorant to do surgery.

and nephritis. We are, therefore, prepared to find our forefathers in Virginia three hundred years ago subject to the same infections, neoplasms and degenerative diseases that beset us today.

These people overate and paid the penalty. A York County jury in 1660 found, after examining a corpse, that "hee died of a surfeit."[3] It is probable that this diagnosis of *colica crapulosa* could mask heart disease then as now. There was much talk of "bellyaches." Dr. George Lee was called on Christmas Eve, 1676, to see Mr. Hill, who "was taken violently Ill wth the bellyake, & could not Stirr out of his bed for 8 or 9 days or thereabouts, & Mr. Lee did administer many things to him, & tooke a great Deale of paines wth him."[4] The historian, Beverley, attributed these bellyaches to dietary indiscretions; but appendicitis, unrecognized as a disease in England until 1812, must have been common and must have exacted its toll.

Seasonings, Cachexes, Fluxes, Scorbutical Dropsies and Gripes make up one writer's imposing list of diseases common in the colony. In the early years "seasoning" was a serious matter. Later, fun was poked at it, though it afforded many physicians a good practice. It was believed that the illness usually experienced by newcomers might be modified or prevented by the proper medical attention, and many masters submitted their new servants to physicians for this treatment.

---

[3] York County Records, v. 3, p. 235.
[4] Surry County Records, v. 2, pp. 107, 108.

"Distemper" was a popular term, occasionally used as if it were a specific disease. It conveniently committed the physician to nothing. Dr. William Irby in 1692 is found in the records "curing Eliza Maybery and her daughter of ye Distemper."[5] Willy Scapes, accounting for his stewardship of one Henry Sewell, writes, "it wear pittey he should goe to Virginia till he be able to manage his owne businesse, for if he should, he would soone lose all he hath gayned, I doubt not but he will gaine more in one yeare now than in two yeares before, he hath beene hitherto verry sickly, he brought a distemper uppon him from Virginia wch hath stuck by him almost all this time, wch was a hardnesse in his boddy wch is now desolved & doth begin to threive."[6]

Epilepsy, the sacred disease of the Hippocratic canon, was called the "falling sickness." In 1686 James Forest of Henrico County obtained exemption from taxation for his son because he was "desperately afflicted with ye Falling Sicknesse soe that he requires continuall Attendance."[7]

In the days when there was no vaccination smallpox was as much a heritage of childhood as measles and mumps are today. The arrival of a new group of slaves from Africa was often the occasion of its introduction into a household or community. There are several references to smallpox in the letters of William Byrd, the elder. In 1686 he wrote a merchant in the Barbadoes that his family was very sick

---

[5]Henrico County Records, v. 5, p. 454.
[6]William and Mary Quarterly, v. 4, p. 171.
[7]Henrico County Records, v. 2, p. 225.

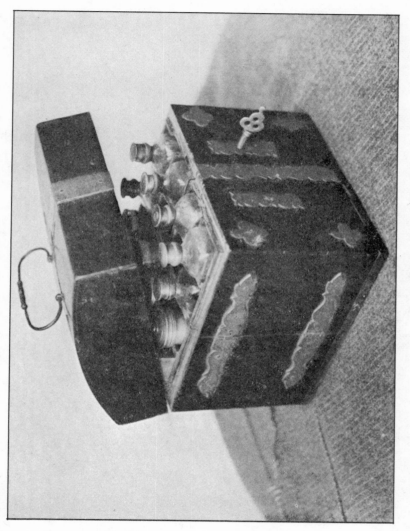

(*Library of the Richmond Academy of Medicine, Miller Collection.*)

Seventeeth Century medicine chest.

with it: "The negroes proved well, but two of them have the Small pox w'h was brought into my family by the Negro's I recd from Gambo." In another letter he wrote, ". . . I have been mighty unhappy in the Negroes by Capt James . . . all yt had ye Small pox (itt seems) hapned into my lott, one dyed on board, & another in ye Boat, my people that went for y'm caught the distemper & brought itt into my family, whereof poor Mrs. Brodnax & 3 of my Negros are allready dead, & abt fifteen more besides my little daughter have them. . . ." Later he added more cheerfully ". . . my family continues yet ill, with the Small pox but (hope in God) the worst is past." Finally he could report that the little daughter "is well recovered & no Signe of them, the worst I hope is past, I made use of Bradlys Doctor & have charg'd a bill on you payable at Sight for 10 lb. . . ."[8]

The common cold made life unhappy, especially during the months of January, February and March. Byrd wrote in 1685, ". . . our little Boy & Molly have been both Sicke wth fever & colds, but are I thanke God now Somewhat better." In 1688 he reported, "I found my wife & children, wth the family (I thank God) Indifferently well, though it hath been a Sickly time here, ever since Xmas, but now blessed bee God all are pretty healthy."[9]

There were isolated cases in Virginia during this century of a contagious disease diagnosed as plague. Whether or

---

[8] Virginia Magazine of History and Biography, v. 25, pp. 134, 136.
[9] Ibid., p. 137.

not this was bubonic plague is open to question. There are also scattered references to scurvy. Cases of violent "ffea-vour & vomiting" and innumerable instances of "fever" are recorded. They must have included a riot of acute diseases such as malaria, dysentery, typhoid and pneumonia.

The death of John Cole in 1691 suggests a train of symptoms similar to those which brought Washington to his grave—*cynanche trachealis,* or inflammatory edema of the larynx. William West, testifying in connection with Cole's death, swore that he "was bedfellow with John Cole . . . when . . . Cole was suddenly seized with a swelling in his throat whereof he Dyed the next day at night when the sd Cole did with as loud a voice as he could speak call unto his Landlord Philip Turpin in these . . . words Philip I am a dead man & I doe give you all that I have in the world. . ."[10]

Besides these sporadic diseases, the Virginia doctor had his hands full with the almost perennial epidemics of measles, smallpox, calenture, bloody flux, winter distempers and possibly plague.

III

Virginia enjoys the reputation of having established at Williamsburg in 1773 the first insane asylum in America. In the Seventeenth Century, however, the barbarous ideas current on the Continent in regard to the management of the insane prevailed here also. The violent were chained or caged, the harmless were allowed at large. These poor

---

[10]Henrico County Records, v. 5, p. 245.

creatures were drugged with camphor, opium or belladonna; purged, vomited and bled; kept in prison and in mechanical restraints, until Philippe Pinel introduced the modern humane treatment. It was late in the Eighteenth Century before the change came.

Early records of the Virginia insane are meagre. Benoni Buck was the first idiot in the colony. In 1637 Ambrose Harmar petitioned the King for the "government" of Benoni, son of the late minister at Jamestown, Richard Buck, "together with his poor estate having had the tuition of him and his brothers for 13 years." The petition was granted after the Governor had certified to Benoni's idiocy. Two years later the idiot was dead, but Governor Harvey wrote the Privy Council imploring "on behalf of the colony that no such grants may pass hereafter, being very prejudicial to the State."[11] In 1661 the commissioners of Surry County contracted with Robert House to board "John Deane an Iddiott," giving him food and clothes and paying his levies. The next year Robert House arrests Thomas Allcock for permitting "John Daines, an Idiott and servant" to go to James Citty, where Allcock gave him strong drink and locked him up in a room with a fire, so that the idiot burned his hand "very sore," costing his master eighty pounds of tobacco for the cure.[12] In 1689 the son of Francis

---

[11]Calendar British State Papers, v. 1574-1660, pp. 251, 294. Mara Buck, Benoni's sister, was apparently also of weak mind. There were several attempts to marry her off, marriage being once regarded as good treatment for insanity.

[12]Surry County Records, v. 1, p. 203.

Redford was exempted from levies because he was an "Idiott."[13]

There are several records of early suicides in Virginia. Dr. Jeremiah Rawlins served on a coroner's jury which found that "ye said Ralph Heaton was imediately before the time of his death a Lunaticke person" and had drowned himself.[14] A citizen testified that on "the 28th of March 1625 Cominge alonge . . . . to the house of Mr. Hugh Crowther, he did see the body of John Verone a servant boye . . . . who had hunge himself w'th an Irone dogg Chaine . . . ." and that "he never hard the boy Complaine of any harde usage . . . but verily beleeveth ye boy willfully hunge himself. . . ."[15] A coroner's jury in 1661 finds that a man servant "hath wilfully cast himself away having viewed diligently According to our Oathes & conscience & hath caused him to be buried at ye next cross path as ye Law Requires wth a stake driven through ye middle of him in his grave hee haveing wilfully Cast himself away."[16] In the same year a York County jury finds that "Walter Catford, who, for want of Grace, tooke a Grindstone and a Roape, and tyed it about his middle and crosse his thighes, and most barbarously went and drowned himselfe contrary to ye law of the king and this country . . . is found guilty of his own death by this Jury. . . ."[17]

---

[13]Henrico County Records, v. 2, p. 300.
[14]Surry County Records, v. 3, p. 347.
[15]Virginia Magazine of History and Biography, v. 23, p. 8.
[16]William and Mary Quarterly, v. 15, p. 181.
[17]Ibid., v. 11, p. 29.

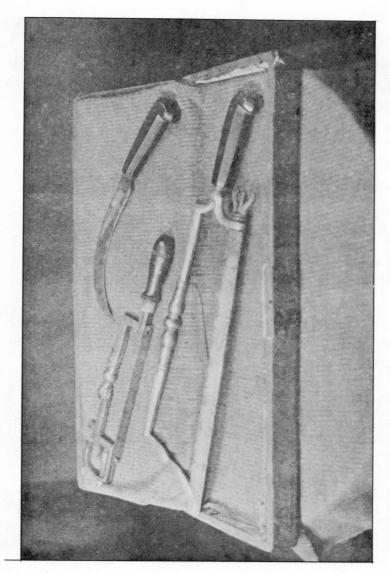

(*Library of the Richmond Academy of Medicine, Miller Collection.*)

Seventeenth Century amputating knife and saws.

The insanity of the defendant in a criminal case is recorded in 1661, when the Court finds "by the discourse of Thomas Cheney that hee is disturbed in his braine, talking wildly and distractedly to such things as are put to him," and orders a suspension of his sentence. He had been convicted of "speaking dangerous and unlawfull words of the kings most Excellent majesty and his Government" and ordered to receive "thirty stripes on his bare back, well layd on till ye blood come, & then returned to ye court."[18] The old belief that insanity was due to yellow and black bile and the heat of dog days was responsible for the faith in restraint and medication, kept up with the hope that the trouble would eventually subside. There is an undercurrent of some such faith in the order of a York County court in 1689: "Whereas John Stock a Madman Liveing in York old feilds whoe keepes running about the neighborhood day and night in a sad Distracted Condition to the great Disturbance of the people, therefore for the prevention of his doeing any future Mischeife It is Ordered by the Court that Mr. Robt. Read, High Sherr: doe take Care that the said Stock bee Lade hold of and safely kept in some close Roome, where hee shall not bee suffered to goe abroad untill hee be in a better condition to Governe himselfe, and that ye said Robert Read is to pvide such helps as may bee Convenient to Looke after him. . . ."[19] However unprepared Virginia was at this time to meet the growing problem of

---

[18]William and Mary Quarterly, v. 11, p. 29.
[19]York County Records, v. 8, p. 363.

her insane, conditions here never reached the extreme that obtained in Vienna, where cases of mental derangement were exhibited in their cells, like animals, for a small fee.

So widespread was the belief at this time in magic, incantations and spells that few minds balked at the grotesque association with medical science of such clairvoyants as Nicholas Culpeper. Englishmen were prepared to hear of almost any sort of strange and wonderful thing in the fairy land of the New World. A communication to the Royal Society of London, containing "observations of luminary emanations from human bodies and from brutes" must have excited the imagination of that learned body. The communication quotes as an example of this strange phenomenon a letter from John Clayton, written at James City, June 23, 1684: "There happened about the month of November to one Madam Susanna Sewall, wife of Major Nic. Sewall, of the Province abovesaid, a strange flashing of sparks (seemed to be of fire) in all the wearing apparel she put one, and so continued till Candlemas. And in the company of several . . . the said Susanna did send several of her wearing apparel, and when they were shaken, it would fly out in sparks, and make a noise, much like unto bay leaves when flung into the fire, and one spark lit on Major Sewall's thumb nail, and there continued at least a minute before it went out, without any heat, all which happened in the company of Wm. Digges. My Lady Baltimore, her mother-in-law, for some time before the death of her son Caecilius Calvert,

had the like happened to her, which has made Madam
Sewall much troubled at what has happened to her. . . ."[20]

IV

Every age has its fashions. In medicine that of the
Seventeenth Century was the clyster.[21] Molière, who always
had a great deal to say about the medicine of his period and
is full of good natured satire, gives an excellent idea of the
prevalence of the clyster habit. In *Monsieur de Pour-
ceaugnac* there is the scene of the unwilling patient fleeing
from pursuing apothecary and doctors, each carrying a
syringe and crying, "It is just a little injection, a little injection, gentle, gentle; it is gentle, gentle: there Sir, take it,
take it; it is to open the bowels." To the perfectly healthy
Jacqueline in *The Physician Inspite of Himself* Molière has
the physician say, "It would not be amiss to bleed you a
little gently, and to administer some little soothing injection." The young lady's objection is over ruled, because,
"It does not matter, the method is salutary." In preserving
the memory of this practice, the fantasy of contemporary
artists has added to the wit of Molière.

The clyster was administered not by the gravity method
but by a large and formidable syringe. The new fashion
was widely advocated and obtained an extraordinary vogue.
Parke states that "Lords and Ladies vied with one another

---

[20]William and Mary Quarterly, v. 1, second series, p. 114.
[21]$\chi\lambda\nu\zeta\epsilon\iota\nu$—to wash away. "Glyster" and "glister" are the usual spell-
ings in the Virginia records.

in belaboring their infarcti and administering enemas."[22]
As a matter of fact the infarctus theory, that fecal impaction
was the cause of all human ills, was not advanced by Johann
Kampf until the next century, when it served simply to
strengthen the universal clyster habit.   Our own century

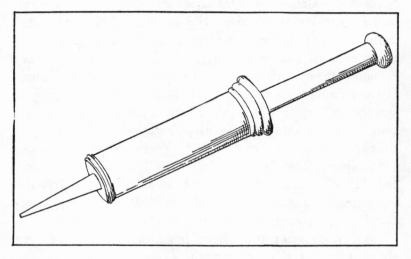

Seventeenth Century Clyster Syringe.

has seen an equally absurd extension of the idea in the
theories of intestinal absorption and autointoxication.

The use of clysters in some form is of course very old.
The ibis is said by Pliny to have demonstrated its use to the

---

[22]Parke: An Epitome of the History of Medicine, p. 201.

Egyptians: "By means of its hooked beak it laves the body through that part."[23]

Two Seventeenth Century authors composed elaborate works on the subject. Regner de Graaf of Holland wrote about it in 1668, and John Arderne two years later published an essay on the clyster and advocated an instrument of his own.

In colonial Virginia, clysters, or "glysters," probably enjoyed the same popularity. There are many references to them in the itemized accounts of doctors, preserved in the county court records. The clyster was apparently administered by the physician, and the fee was thirty pounds of tobacco. Among the effects of Nathaniel Hill was "1 old syringe."[24] In York County records we find that Thomas Whitehead in 1660 paid Edmond Smith for "2 glysters."[25] George Wale's account to the estate of Thomas Baxter in 1658 included a similar charge.[26] George Light in 1657 paid Dr. Modé fifty pounds of tobacco for "a glister and Administering."[27] John Clulo, Francis Haddon and William Lee each prosecuted bills for similar services.

From the "hiera" of Rufus of Ephesus to the present time purgation has been the strong fort of therapy. According to an old saying:

---

[23]Pliny, Book II, ch. 41.
[24]Henrico County Records, v. 5, p. 182.
[25]York County Records, v. 3, p. 212.
[26]Ibid., p. 67.
[27]Ibid., v. 2, p. 69.

"Know in beginning of all sharpe diseases,
'Tis counted best to make evacuation."

The Seventeenth Century was no exception, and we find
Virginia physicians prescribing the purge with lavish frequency. Francis Haddon in 1660 prescribed for one patient
a purging "Bolus," purging clyster and purging pills, and
charged thirty pounds of tobacco; for another patient, two
purges and two purging "electuaries," for 140 pounds of
tobacco.[28] Dr. Giles Modé in 1657 prescribed a laxative
syrup, for twenty pounds of tobacco.[29] Daniel Parke in
1665 asked eighty pounds of tobacco for two purges.[30]
Dr. George Wale prescribed "2 potions of torrefyed
Rubub" and "2 potions of Rubarb and mirab." and charged
160 pounds of tobacco.[31] Dr. John Clulo received thirty-six
pounds each for two "purging potions."[32] Dr. Jeremiah
Rawlins charged 150 pounds of tobacco for three "purges
Rhubarb mirabolus."[33] George Eland in 1697 was paid
handsomely for the "pfluxinge of Emanuell Dil a Seaman."[34]

Evidence of the importance which physicians have always
attached to purgation is the fact that the first medical book
ever printed was a *Laxierkalendar* in 1457. There was a
great deal of nonsense connected with the giving of purges,

---

[28]York County Records, v. 3, p. 203; v. 4, p. 442.
[29]Ibid., v. 2, p. 69.
[30]Ibid., v. 4, p. 57.
[31]Ibid., v. 3. p. 67.
[32]Ibid., p. 66.
[33]Ibid., p. 259.
[34]Elizabeth City County Records, v. 1684-99, p. 143.

which continued well into the Seventeenth Century. Reliance
was still placed on the horoscope, and medical practice had
not entirely got away from the purgation calendars of the
Middle Ages, which indicated under each sign of the zodiac
the proper time to administer the cathartic and often fore-
cast awful happenings that were to befall humanity under
the various planetary conjunctions. In spite of the reck-
less therapy of the age there was at least one sane contemporary author and teacher, Francis Sylvius of Leyden
(1614-1672). He may have taught the few Virginia doctors who were educated in Holland. In his *Praxeos
Medicae Liber Quartus,* translated and published in London,
1682, he states: "For it may happen to Infants as to people
of years, that all are not alike easily, speedily or largely
purged by any Medicine. For which cause, lest they should
get harm by a strong Medicine, it is better to give a gentle
Purge at several times, and that a little at a time, rather
than together and at once. For a Physician cannot be too
cautious."

V

Phlebotomy was another therapeutic sheet anchor which
enjoyed wide popularity during this century. It was a very
ancient method and its efficacy was as yet unquestioned by
most physicians. There was hardly a disease for which it
was not used. Sydenham during the Seventeenth Century
in England employed it in practically every disorder, though
he was more moderate than some of his contemporaries.

There was always, however, some stigma connected with it.
In the Middle Ages medicine was largely in the hands of
the clergy, who regarded bloodletting, surgery and dissection as phases of medicine to be farmed out to the more
menial barbers and barber-surgeons. Bloodletting was,
therefore, more particularly the function of the chirurgeon
or barber. It will be recalled that Washington in his last
illness had himself bled by his overseer before sending for
a physician, indicating the menial character of the procedure.
This does not mean that phlebotomy did not become a
highly technical process, or that physicians did not resort to
it. Every physician carried his lancet, and bleeding glasses
were often costly and were handed down as family heir-
looms. It was an old saying:

"By bleeding, to the marrow commeth heat,
  It maketh cleane your braine, relieves your eye,
  It mends your appetite, restoreth sleepe,
  Correcting humours that do waking keepe:
  All inward parts and senses also clearing,
  It mends the voyce, touch, smell & tast, & hearing."

The rationale of the procedure varied. The individual
might be phlethoric, his blood overheated or the scene of
"morbific matter" which needed to be evacuated. Thus
developed the theory that the vein must be opened "corre-
sponding to the particular part affected and its emunctory
or excretory channel." The Hippocratic method held sway
for many hundred years. It was known as the "derivative"
method and consisted in bleeding the patient freely on the

side of the lesion. With the ascendency of Arabian medicine about 900 A. D. the so-called "revulsive" method came into vogue. This consisted in less heroic bleeding on the side opposite the lesion. Brissot (1478-1522) ably took a stand for the return to the derivative method, which became the practice in the Seventeenth Century. Bleeding was usually heroic. Some idea of its extent is obtained from the experiences cited by Guy Patin, who twelve times bled his wife, twenty times his son and seven times himself. M. Cousinot bled a case of rheumatism sixty-four times. The procedure was not considered effective unless the patient became unconscious. "Bleed until syncope" was the slogan. Copious draughts of water constituted an essential part of the technique. Well into the Seventeenth Century the horoscope was used to determine the proper time for bleeding.

The Virginia court records show the phlebotomy practice in full sway here. Dr. Modé's bill to George Light includes "a phlebothany to Jno Simonds" and "a phlebothany to yr mayd."[35] Dr. Henry Power twice bled Thomas Cowell of York County in 1680,[36] and Patrick Napier twice phlebotomized "Allen Jarves, deceased" "in the cure of a cancer of his mouth."[37] Colonel Daniel Parke in 1665 rendered John Horsington a bill for "lettinge blood" from his servant;[38] and we find Dr. Jeremiah Rawlins and Francis Haddon engaging in the same practice.

---

[35] York County Records, v. 2, p. 69.
[36] Ibid., v. 6, p. 330.
[37] Ibid., v. 4, p. 144.
[38] Ibid., v. 4, p. 67.

VI

Cupping, which is as old as the animal horn with which it was executed by primitive peoples, was commonly resorted to.   Dr. Francis Haddon charged twenty pounds of tobacco for cupping a man in 1660.[39]   In the Northampton records there is a deposition of Dr. John Severne to the effect that eight days after Mr. Walker's boy was whipped, "he being a chirurgeon was requested to take a view and to look upon him the sd boy beinge sicke, and this depont supposinge that cuppinge would do him good, hee this depont did cupp him. . . ."[40]

Among other popular therapeutic procedures were vomiting, sweating and blistering.   A well known lampoon connected with the name of Dr. John Lettsom of London, who took a peculiar interest in American medicine in the next century, runs:

> "I, John Lettsom
> Blisters, bleeds and sweats 'em.
> If after that they please to die
> I John Lettsom."

True to the spirit of the times we find Dr. Giles Modé prescribing in 1657 "an electuary with vomiting."[41]   In the Henrico Records there is a deposition that Dr. Irby came to Mr. Mayberrie's house "to visit the sd Mayberries Wife

---

[39]York County Records, v. 3, p. 203.
[40]Northampton County Records, v. 1640-45, p. 18.
[41]York County Records, v. 2, p. 69.

& Daughter whome he had then under Cure & asking how they did she said I and my Daughter are rather worse than better by what we took off you, & the sd Irby replied he had brought some sweating medicines purposely for them in his Pocket. . . ."[42]

VII

From time immemorial the urine has been naturally the subject of medical interest. Actuarius as early as 600 A. D. invented a graduate for measuring the urine, and Avicenna is said to have discovered its sweet taste in diabetes. Van Helmont in the late Sixteenth Century actually weighed twenty-four hour specimens and was a pioneer in the gravimetric method of urinalysis. The presence of albumen, the nature of sediments, and the information to be derived from microscopic study were not dreamt of in the Seventeenth Century.

Urine examination as practised in this century was usually of an entirely different nature. It was known as Uroscopy, or "water casting." The urine, usually in a flask, was brought to the physician, who held it to the light with solemn and judicial air, while he read the patient's fate in the uplifted urinal. Anyone who has visited the art galleries of Amsterdam and the Hague must have been impressed by the frequency with which uroscopy was the subject of the Dutch painters. Solemnly the physician diagnoses Mal d'Amour. The urinal became the emblem on the signboard

---

[42]Henrico County Records, v. 5, p. 454.

of the mediaeval physician. Molière's *Flying Doctor* depicts the Seventeenth Century physician engaged in a urinalysis: "This urine shows a great deal of heat, a great inflammation of the bowels; it is, however, not so very bad."

"Gorgibus—'Eh, What-Sir, are you swallowing it?'

"Scanarelle—'Do not be surprised at that, doctors, as a rule, are satisfied with looking at it; but I am a doctor out of the common, I swallow it, for by tasting it I discern much better the cause and the effect of the disease. But, to tell you the truth, there was too little to judge by; let her make water again!'"

The Reverend John Clayton's letter from Virginia to the Royal Society refers to his method of urinalysis. The parson, who was apparently practising medicine on a parity with regular physicians, had a scientific mind and was not a uroscopist or urine gazer of the ordinary variety. He says, "I had Glasses blown would hold about five Ounces, others about ten Ounces, with Necks so small, that a Drop would make a considerable Variation; with these I could make much more critical and satisfactory Observations as to the specifical Gravity of Liquors, having critical Scales, than by any other Way yet by me tried. I use this Method to weigh Urines, which Practice I would recommend to the inquisitive and critical Physicians. I had made many Observations hereof, but all Notes were likewise lost with my other things. Yet I have begun afresh; for there are more signal Variations in the Weights of Urines than one would at first imagine; and when the Eye can discover little, but judge two

Urines to be alike, they may be found to differ very much as to Weight. By Weight I find Observations may be made of Affections in the Head, which rarely make any visible Alterations in the Urine. I have found two Urines not much unlike differ two and twenty Grains in the Quantity of about four or five Ounces: But let them that make these Essays weigh all their Urines when cold, lest they be thereby deceived."[43]

The average Seventeenth Century physician tried to over-awe his patients with "long tirades of technical drivel." He certainly could not overawe them with mechanical equip-ment. He had no stethoscope or sphygmomanometer. Even the clinical thermometer was known only to such pioneering inventive minds as Sanctorius. We may be sure, however, that he felt the pulse and looked wise in doing so. There was still great faith in deductions from palpation of the radial artery. The pulse lore of the century was tre-mendous in amount. The fantastic theories of Galen, who wrote sixteen books on the subject and described a pulse for every disease, were still current. Dutch artists of the century have left striking canvases showing the doctor in the act of taking the pulse. The watch, which has become such a familiar accessory, is lacking in these paintings. One of the earliest records of a watch in Virginia dates back to 1660, in which year an attachment was granted to Captain Ellyson, executor of Dr. Henry Waldron's estate, against

---

[43]Force: Tracts, v. 3, "Letter of Rev. John Clayton."

Thomas Bowles for three pounds sterling for a watch of Waldron's which Bowles had carried to England and sold.[44] At least one Seventeenth Century Virginia doctor owned a watch.

VIII

It is difficult to appreciate how different was the surgery practised in the Seventeenth Century from that with which we are familiar today.   Asepsis was still waiting for bacteriology, and anesthesia was a dream to be first realized in America in 1842.   The head and chest were sacrosanct. None but a fool dared invade the abdomen.   Lithotomy was proscribed by the Hippocratic oath, though many submitted to the lithotomist's knife and, like Pepys, lived to celebrate the occasion.   As William Clowes, the best of the Elizabethan surgeons, said, "This sort of dangerous business was chiefly practised by wandering cataract couchers, lithotomists, herniotomists and booth surgeons."   A few daring surgeons had successfully performed Caesarean sections, ovariotomy, lithotomy, urethrotomy and herniotomy, had operated for fistula and cataract, and had made a good beginning in plastic surgery, but the average surgeon's business was chiefly concerned with wounds, fractures, dislocations, amputations, abscesses and ulcers.   Minor surgery, especially phlebotomy, was usually left to the barbers.

---

[44]York County Records, v. 3, p. 261.   (Standard: Colonial Virginia, p. 211, gives 1697 as the first record of a watch in Virginia.   Two watches are mentioned in Rich. Wake's Inventory, 1648; one in Thos. Fawn's will, 1651.)

A fair appraisal of early Virginia surgery is difficult. The distinction between doctor and surgeon was not as sharp as it was in Europe. In general the difference was one of superior education and training rather than of specialization in practice. Colonial surgery was neither fish, flesh nor fowl. It had lost, certainly in Virginia, its tonsorial functions and gained little in their stead; and since it now shared with the physician the business of phlebotomy its only recourse was to meddle with drugs. We find surgeons throughout the Virginia records prescribing medicine with about the same frequency as did the doctors.

The early records in regard to surgery are concerned chiefly with the treatment of wounds, burns, frostbite, fractures, dislocations and ulcers. The York County records show several surgeons at work. Dr. Haddon's treatment of an amputation was to give two cordials on the day of the operation and a purge four days later, with frequent ointments and external applications. After two months it became necessary to bleed the patient. Haddon's effects contained a dismembering saw.[45]

Dr. Robert Ellyson in 1661 testified that "Fortune Perkins came to my house about Whitsuntide last being sorely bruised in his body about the Armes and sides and one of his shoulders dislocated which was by mee reduced but how it came I know not. . . . For the said cure I doe demand sattisfaccon six hundred pounds of tobaccoe and referre it to

[45]York County Records, v. 4, p. 442; v. 5, pp. 196-98.

consideration. . . ."[46] In the year 1689 judgment was
granted Dr. Richard Starke "agt Hugh Norrell for 3 lb
sterl for the pfecting of a cure of a dangerous wound in
Edward Maylin's head, which was committed by the said
Norrell and itt appearing . . . that the said Starke was
Imployed therein by the said Norrell. . . ."[47] In the Surry
County records we find that Miles Berriffe is ordered to pay
five pounds sterling to Dr. Thomas Watkinson "for his care
pains and cure of his the said Berriffe's will full wound in
his throat with costs."[48]

Sores of the feet and legs are frequently mentioned and
were probably due to the custom of going barefoot. They
must have been a form of impetigo. The following deposition was made by Dr. Henry Blagrave in Dr. Patrick
Napier's suit against Ralph Graves: "Mrs. Graves having
a concarous ulcer in her Instepp with other internall distempers sent for mee I coming there found Mr. Napier with
whom having had some conference . . . and finding his wants
of some necessary medycines . . . offered him any I had by
mee. . . ." When Blagrave next went to visit Mrs. Graves
he found that Napier had not used the medicines and so
"my credit being concerned by my former applicacon . . .
did make it my businesse to wayt upon hir till shee was
pfectly cured and recovered."[49]

Dr. John Holloway is mentioned for a cure of John

[46]York County Records, v. 3, p. 329.
[47]Ibid., v. 8, p. 367.
[48]Surry County Records, v. 6, p. 230.
[49]York County Records, v. 3, p. 376.

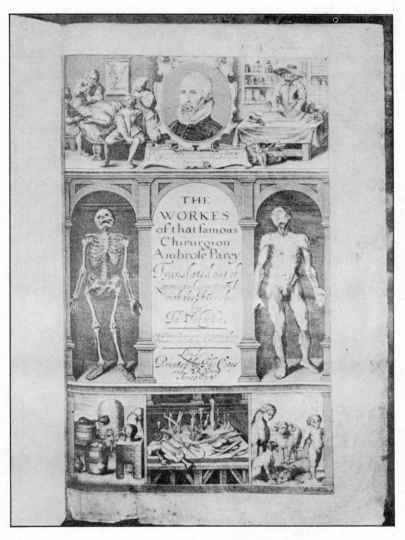

Title page of the Works of Paré, a medical book often found in
Seventeenth Century Virginia libraries.

Hatnall's ulcer of the throat in 1637.[50] Dr. John Severne
in 1640 treated Anne Moye for "a tumor in her neck with
inflamacon of the Amiddalls of her throate."[51] Alexander
Meckeny cured "the scald head" of young Thomas
Brookes.[52] Dr. William Irby in 1684 rendered a bill for
setting "ye sd Knibbs sons thigh."[53] William Townsend
described his services as "attendance in surgery."[54] Samuel
Tracy in 1661 undertook the cure of a servant's leg and
later had a patient whose complaint was "pain and
bruises."[55]

Surgeons were occasionally called upon to care for victims
of the duel, which was common enough at that time. George
Harrison's death from a simple cut in the knee, received in
a duel in 1624, did not speak well for his surgical at-
tendant.[56]

Compared to the formidable array of surgical implements
in contemporary texts the armamentarium of the Virginia
chirurgeon was simple indeed. There are bare records of
surgical chests containing instruments, clyster syringes,
basins, galli-pots and salvatories. Dr. John Holloway's will
left "a chest of instruments and lancets," and his inventory

---

[50]Northampton County Records, v. 1632-40, p. 85.
[51]Ibid., v. 1640-45, p. 174.
[52]Henrico County Records, v. 3, p. 33.
[53]Ibid., v. 2, p. 170.
[54]York County Records, v. 8, p. 50.
[55]Ibid., v. 3, pp. 321, 325.
[56]Calendar British State Papers, v. 1574-1660, p. 61. It is stated in
the Virginia Magazine of History and Biography, v. 1, p. 347, that from
the time of the Company down to the Revolution "there is no record of any
duel in Virginia."

showed "1 Playster box of instruments, some other instruments" and "1 case of Lancettes."[57]   Andrew Winter's will, 1697, disposed of "a case of instruments & salvatory & case of lancets."[58]   Dr. Waldron left "a chest of physical meanes."[59]   The estate of Dr. Richard Starke included "Medson Book and instruments" valued at thirteen pounds sterling.   The inventory of Richard Crashaw, 1677, includes "2 Surgeons instruments of silver" valued at four shillings.[60] Dr. Henry Lee's son, dying in 1693, had among his effects "a Chirurgeons box" which he had evidently inherited from his father.[61]

To understand properly the Seventeenth Century practice of medicine in Virginia one must visualize the doctor and chirurgeon practising side by side, often confused with one another, with no clearly defined differentiation unless it were one of education.   There were no obstetricians, only midwives; no dentists, except perhaps an occasional travelling one, the emergency dentistry being in the hands of the physicians; no specialists to bewilder the public.   Neurologists, pediatricians, otolaryngologists, gynecologists, pathologists and the like did not exist.

---

[57]Northampton County Records, v. 1640-45, pp. 257-59.
[58]York County Records, v. 6, p. 171.
[59]Ibid., v. 3, p. 18.
[60]Virginia Magazine of History and Biography, v. 33, p. 27.
[61]William and Mary Quarterly, v. 24, p. 48.

CHAPTER VI

HOUSING THE SICK

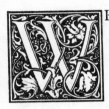HEN we think of the rise of hospitals in America we naturally have in mind as the first the Pennsylvania Hospital, founded in 1750 in Philadelphia under the fostering influence of Dr. Thomas Bond and Benjamin Franklin. A little later, in 1769, the New York Hospital was started by Dr. Peter Middleton, John Jones and Samuel Bard.[1]

One hundred and fifty years before either of these hospitals was thought of, interesting beginnings had been made in the colony of Virginia in the housing of the sick and wounded. The first hospital built in Virginia, as well as the first built in America, was constructed in 1612 in a new town near the Falls of James River, called Henricopolis. Early in September 1611 Sir Thomas Dale had proceeded fifty miles up the river from James City and had laid out

---

[1] Hospitals were an outgrowth of Christianity, and their rise was one of the bright spots of the Middle Ages. The movement was forwarded by Helena, mother of Constantine (335 A. D.). Many large and remarkable institutions sprang up over Europe. Until the Thirteenth Century the hospitals were entirely under the care of the church. Then municipalities began to take them over. In England St. Bartholomews was founded in 1137, Holy Cross (Winchester) in 1132, St. Mary's in 1197, St. Thomas's in 1212. The first hospital in the New World was erected by Cortez in the city of Mexica in 1524. In 1639 a Hotel Dieu was established in Canada by the Duchesse d'Aguilon, and ultimately located in Quebec. "The first hospital in what is now the United States was established on Manhattan Island in 1663." (Garrison: History of Medicine.)

the new town. The site is the present Dutch Gap. Here
one of the best towns in the colony was soon prospering.
It was traversed by three streets faced with well framed
houses. It had a handsome wooden church and a stately
brick one in the making. There were store houses, watch
houses and block houses, and the whole was strongly impaled. Across the river, also impaled and guarded by block
houses, was the hospital. It was designed to accommodate
eighty patients. Beds were on hand before the building was
complete. Provision was made for both medical and surgical patients, and nurses were in readiness to minister to the
suffering. Hamor speaks of the hospital as "Mount malado
(a retreat or guest house for sicke people, a high seat and
wholesome air). . . ."[2] From another contemporary observer we learn that "Here they were building also an
Hospitall with fourescore lodgings (and beds alreadie sent
to furnish them) for the sicke and lame, with keepers to attend them for their comfort and recoverie."[3] We hear
nothing more of this hospital. It was doubtless burned in
the general conflagration accompanying the massacre of
1622.

In 1620 "a charter of orders for the better preserving
and nourishing of the emigrants" was issued by the London
Company. It provided "that . . . the people now sent, and
which hereafter shall come, may be the better provided
against . . . sicknesse, (seeing in the health of the people

[2]Brown: First Republic, p. 209.
[3]Force: Tracts, v. 1, "New Life of Virginea," pp. 13, 14.

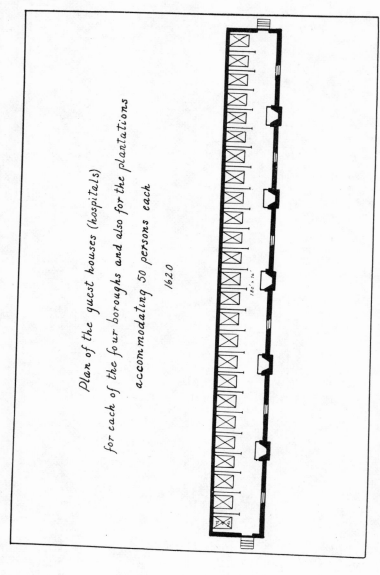

Plan of the hospitals designed in 1620 for the four boroughs of the Virginia colony.

consisteth the very life, strenth, increase and prosperity of the whole general colony) . . . : First, in each of the four ancient general Boroughs . . . as also in each of the particular Plantations, a Guest-house [hospital] shall be built for the lodging and entertaining of fifty persons in each, upon their first arrival. Said houses to be raised in wholesome places, each shall be 16 feet broad within, and 180 feet long . . . with 25 beds of four foot broad, six foot long, and two foot height from the ground in equal distances and with partitions of boards between: Five conveniently placed Chimnies for fire, and sufficient windows for wholesomeness of air."[4] Three years later the Privy Council ordered "Guest houses to be built for harboring sick men and receiving strangers."[5] There are many reasons why the institutional care of the sick was thus so specifically provided for. There were few women in the colony, great poverty prevailed, and sickness was widespread and fatal. With public granaries and public ownership of land a real communism existed, and the guest house was a form of social service which naturally grew out of it. With the dissolution of the Company these hospitals disappeared.

---

[4]Brown: First Republic, pp. 377, 378. Note that two patients were expected to occupy one bed, 25 beds being provided for 50 persons. The custom of crowding many persons into one sleeping apartment is mentioned by the Marquis de Chastellux, who was in Virginia 150 years later. Haggard, in *Devils, Drugs and Doctors,* quotes Max Nordau as saying of the Hotel Dieu: "In one bed of moderate width lay four, five, or six sick persons beside each other, the feet of one to the head of another; children beside gray-haired old men; indeed, incredible but true, men and women intermingled together."

[5]Ibid., p. 543.

There was little standing on ceremony in those days. When help was needed, strangers approached strangers with frontier freedom. Inns were poor and expensive. The traveler passed them by to knock at the first house and ask a night's lodging. Whether he was a pleasure or a burden he was accommodated, perhaps in the one room shared by all the family. Beauchamp Plantagenet, who traveled in Virginia in 1648, declared that there was "free quarter everywhere," and Beverley early in the next century writes that "poor planters who have but one bed will very often sit up or lie upon a form or couch all night to make room for a weary traveller." Out of such hospitality arose the custom of housing the sick in private homes.

There is much evidence in the county records to show that private hospitalization of the sick was common and that each physician probably took care of a few patients in his own house when the seriousness of the illness, the distance from the doctor or other factors peculiar to that day and time made it necessary. One of the most interesting court records of Surry County describes how in 1676 Dr. George Lee was most reluctantly forced to take Mrs. Richard Hill into his house for medical care. In the record Dr. Lee's servant testifies that Mrs. Hill's husband "sending to Mr. Lee for a rich Cordiall for his Wife & alsoe yor depont [deponent] to come to her, & accordingly Mr. Lee & yor depont found her in a very weake condicion, with a violent ffeavour & vomiting & very big with child . . . and by her Earnest request to Mr. Lee & me he stayed with her two nights &

days, administred Severall things to her, & yor depont
stayed three nights and days . . . she . . . begging and
Intreating Mr. Lee to Lett her come into his house to lye
in at, or Else shee should be a dead woman . . . for in that
house . . . where shee dwelt shee would be starved wth Cold,
it being such an open house, & besides shee had not anything
to Eate but an old Sow, & that shee should perish & dye &
her life was more to her than all the world, to wch Mr. Lee
made her answere her house might be made warmer & she
might send to her neighbours to gett poultry . . . for he had
noe accomodation for her Neither would he take any such
trouble upon him, for he had but one roome wch was ffitting
for any such use, and yt he lay in himselfe & he would not
turne himselfe out of it for anybody in Virg^a, besides he
dayly Expected his wife in . . . shee replyed yt shee knew
the roome very well, & it was bigg Enough for himselfe his
wife & her to, soe by her vehemt Impertuneing Mr. Lee he
told her . . . when her feavour & vomiting was gon & yt shee
was in a condicon to be removed he would come down & discourse wth her & her Husband about it, & soe Mr. Lee went
home. . . ." The deposition goes on to explain that the next
day Mrs. Hill forced her servants and maid to carry her in
her boat to Mr. Lee's landing, and she and her maid then
took up their residence at the doctor's house. Several days
later the husband also came there and seemed pleased with
the arrangement, although Mr. Lee explained that it was
against his will and that "shee would be continually takeing
of medicines if Mr. Lee would administer them to her,

whilst if he would have administered them to her as fast as shee would have them the charge would amount to more than he was willing to pay, Mr. Hill replyed he could not help it, shee will have her humour . . . & I will see you paid." Mr. Hill stayed on, and "on Christmas Eve the sd Mr. Hill . . . was taken violently Ill wth the belly ake, & could not Stirr out of his bed for 8 or 9 Days or thereabouts, & Mr. Lee did administer many things to him, & tooke a great Deale of paines wth him. . . ." The record then describes at length the lying-in of Mrs. Hill, the climax of the story being that Mr. Hill refused to pay the bill, and Dr. Lee was compelled to bring suit to collect his fee.[6]

This was not an isolated case. Dr. George Eland, of Elizabeth City County, testified in court in 1695 that Edward Limington of Pennsylvania, "after being at my house some few dayes did there dye & was buryed in my Orchard & yt Nathaniel Hinson Mercht of ye Shipp who ye said Limington came with had marryed ye Governor's daughter of Pennsylvania & withall gave me ye sd Eland a great charge of him but it was soe ordered hee Dyed as aforementioned."[7]

In York County we find "Captain Stephen Gill the Chirurgion" filing a bill in 1645 against the estate of Henry Brooke, merchant, for one thousand pounds of tobacco "for Diett, lodging, phissicke and attendance . . . in the tyme of

[6]Surry County Records, v. 2, pp. 107, 108.
[7]Elizabeth City County Records, v. 1684-99, p. 357.

his sicknesse."[8]   George Wale, also of York, in 1659 secured an attachment against the estate of Thomas Page
"for physick, Dyett, trouble and other chardges in his sickness & for burying him. . . ."[9]

The Vestry Book of Christ Church Parish gives several
instances of the housing of the sick by physicians.   In 1681
William Poole, Chirurgeon, was paid a thousand pounds of
tobacco by order of the vestry "for keeping one Mary
Teston, poore impotent pson."   Two years later the parish
sent him another patient, the conditions of whose payment
are interesting.   On July 20, 1683, "It is ordered by this
present Vestry that Dr. William Poole take home to his
house the pson of Christopher Goulder of this parish, and
use the utmost of his endeavor to Cure him of his Blindness, and in Case that Dor. Poole Should make a Cure
thereof, then the Said Dor. Poole is to have, for the Cure
Two Thousand pounds of Tobacco & Cask, But in Case the
Doctor not cure ye Said Christopr Goulder, that then the
Said Dor Poole is to have but Reasonble Satisfaction for
his Trouble."[10]   In 1689 the same vestry book records the
payment of a thousand pounds of tobacco to Dr. Robert
Boodle for keeping Bridget Press, "a poore Decripped &
lame woman" for twelve months.[11]   Dr. Boodle was also
paid a thousand pounds for keeping "William Stone a poore
Decripped and Ulserated man."

---

[8]York County Records, v. 2, p. 88.
[9]Ibid., v. 3, p. 181.
[10]Vestry Book. Christ Church, Middlesex County, pp. 34, 38.
[11]Ibid., pp. 40, 60, 64. 67.

In Rappahannock County in 1674 there is a deposition by John Stringer, Chirurgeon, that "William Stoakes lying sicke at yr deponts [deponent's] house he your deponent ... asked the sd Stoakes if it pleased God to take him out of this world ... how will [you] dispose of your bills. ...."[12] In Northampton County "It is ordered in consideracon of John Holloways neglect in the cure of Thomas Wignall that the said Hollowaye shall take Wignall home and keep him accordinge to his promise, and use to doe his best indever in the cure of his legge."[13]   Another instance of this custom is that of the illustrious rebel, Nathaniel Bacon, who was taken, a sick man, to the house of Dr. Pate in Gloucester County.   There dysentery caused his death and saved him from the noose of the revengeful Berkeley.   Some accounts say that he died at the house of Dr. Green, but the Commissioners sent from England to investigate the rebellion reported that "Hee lay sick at one Mr. Pates in Gloster County of the Bloody Flux, and (as Mr. Pate himself affirms) accompanyed with a Lousy Disease. ...."[14]

There is a good deal of evidence that the sick were not infrequently cared for in the houses of men and women who were not doctors, but who probably had acquired some reputation for nursing, and who found the business profitable. In Rappahannock County, 1686, James Stanford is granted 1,200 pounds of tobacco against the estate of Nathaniel

---

[12]Rappahannock County Records, v. 3, p. 77.
[13]Northampton County Records, v. 1632-40, p. 128.
[14]Virginia Magazine of History and Biography, v. 4, p. 153.

Gubb "in Recompence for his Care and the trouble of his house in the time of the sd Mr. Gubbs sickness. . ."[15] The same year Stephen Bendrick agrees to provide "wholesome dyett, washing & Lodging" for Robert Holmes, who was "afflicted with lameness and sickness," and also for his two daughters; and to "convey him with all expedicon . . . to the Potomack to the doctor Arnold for his Care . . . .," and to pay all his debts, in consideration for the grant of Holmes' plantation and dwelling house.[16] Again, in Richmond County we find Thomas Tippitt, "having taken care of a servant woman belonging to Den McCarty named Sarah Banbury during her Child birth," receiving 400 pounds of tobacco from McCarty "in full satisfaction for his sd care."[17] Finally, in 1670, there is the account in the York records of Theophilus Brown "comeing to the said Overstreete's house very sick" and promising that if he died he would give Overstreete three barrels of corn and one cow.[18]

---

[15]Rappahannock County Records, v. 11, p. 18.
[16]Ibid., v. 8, p. 322.
[17]Richmond County Records, v. 1, part 2, p. 30.
[18]York County Records, v. 4, p. 435.

CHAPTER VII

WOMEN AND MEDICINE

I

Nurses

T was 1836 before Theodor Friedner opened at Kaiserworth the first school for deaconesses; 1860 before Miss Nightingale set about teaching the first English trained nurses at St. Thomas's; 1873 before a trained nurse was produced in America; and 1886 before Virginia joined the movement. In Europe the Seventeenth Century was the dark age of nursing, and the care of the sick sank as low as the hospitals in which it was practised. Conditions were little changed two hundred years later, when Dickens immortalized Sairey Gamp. She, with her pawky umbrella and talk of the hypothetical Mrs. Harris, was a type of the "pudgy, slatternly, dowdy looking female, of drunken and dubious habits" who was the nurse of that day. Her counterpart was to be found in France in the sisters, Mme. Pochet and Mme. Gibou.

In Virginia conditions were probably better, for there were none of the great municipal hospitals to corrupt both the manners and morals of the nursing profession. We encounter nurses early in Virginia history. In 1612 the hospital at Henricopolis was supplied with "keepers" to attend

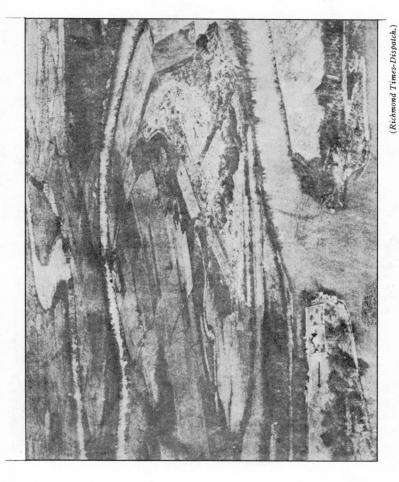

(Richmond Times-Dispatch.)

Site of Henricopolis from the air. The arrow points to the bank on which the hospital stood.

the sick and wounded. These were probably male nurses. While Sisters of Charity ministered to the sick on the Continent, all the English military hospitals used soldiers for nurses until the middle of the Nineteenth Century. It is unlikely that an English frontier hospital would have had women as nurses. For many years after 1607 women were scarce in the colony. It was 1620 before the *Jonathan,* with almost two hundred maids for wives, and the *London Merchant,* with still more, arrived to meet the deficiency.

During the rest of the century we find references to both male and female nurses, although male ones were apparently more common. Charles Donne's name occurs frequently in the York records, and in 1658 he asked 1,100 pounds of tobacco from the estate of John Golney for "attendance in sickness 11 weeks, dyett, washing and other accomodation."[1] John Lacey in 1688 left all of his estate, except two cows, "to Mary Cawley and Agnes Rogers p'sons yt I have made Choice of to looke after me in the time of my sicknesse."[2] In 1683 Robert Evans was paid 100 pounds of tobacco for his care of "a poor aged man" who "lay some small time sick at his house. . . ."[3] An interesting example of a verbal will, as well as of the care of the sick, appears in the Henrico records for 1689: "Tho Watts late dec'd did for ye trouble & charge Jno. Cressy was at in ye time of his sicknesse give & verbally bequeath unto ye sd Cressy all his estate both

---

[1]York County Records, v. 3, p. 67.
[2]Ibid., v. 8, p. 227.
[3]Henrico County Records, v. 2, p. 153.

real and personal he ye sd Cressy paying all just demands against ye same. . . ."[4]

These nurses were of course self constituted and often combined other occupations with that of caring for the sick. The men frequently acted as undertakers. Peter Butts was paid 500 pounds of tobacco in 1677, "being for his trouble & paines with him in his sicknesse & for funerall charges."[5] Several years later John Hunt was awarded two cows in part payment when he petitioned the court "that he hath beene att a great charge and troble with Henry Todd whoe was mortally wounded by a negro, by keeping him and dressing his wounds and alsoe buryeing him. . ."[6] Edward Thomas's bill to the estate of James Drake reads:

	£	s.	d.

"To my wife and selfe attending of him in ye time
  of his sicknesse and the trouble of my house. . 1-10-00
To a winding sheet. 0-12-00
To a coffing for him, as being his desire to
  have one. 0-12-00
To ffunerall Charges and Trouble. . . . . .1-00-00"[7]

An account of the expenses and money "layd out by Thomas Batts for Eliz. Jenkins in ye time of her Sickness by ye sd Jenkins request & order" in 1693 included:

"To 2 gallons of rume at 40 p galln. . . . . . . 80 (pounds
To 6 lb. sugar at 6d p lb. . . . . 36 tobacco)

4Henrico County Records, v. 5, p. 105.
5York County Records, v. 6, p. 20.
6Ibid., v. 7, p. 199.
7Ibid., v. 8, p. 237.

To 2 ... of Strong Beere.............. 07
To ffetching her coffin & buriall.........100
To ye trouble of my house..............100
To washing & Lodginge................050
To ffowles.........................050
To candles Expended & watching in time of
   her sickness......................100"[8]

George Woodward's bill to William Hukins included:

"p : 5 months Diett for his wife.........500 (pounds
 p : the charge Lyeinge in & sick.........300 tobacco)
 p : the charge of Buriall & a sheete......200
                                          ————
                                          1000"[9]

The county records are full of similar charges. It was
a day of mourning rings, black gloves, ribbons, scarfing and
sitting up with the corps, and funerals were elaborate affairs
celebrated by the firing of guns, feasting, drinking and
carousal. Debts for the funeral of Mrs. Elizabeth Epes,
who died in 1678, included:

"To 10 lb. Butter..................... 50 (pounds
To 2 Galls. Brandy................... 70 tobacco)
To ½ Pepper, ½ of Ginger........... 9
To 5 Gals. wine.....................150
To 8 lb. Sugar..................... 32

[8]Elizabeth City County Records, v. 1684-99.
[9]Surry County Records, v. 1, p. 92.

To 1 Steer of 7 years.................600
To 3 large weathers.................450
                                    ────
                                    1361"[10]

Ralph Langley, "being very weak & Crazie," concludes his
will in 1683 with a mild protest against such excesses: "I
beseech yr honor that there be noe more charge at my
funerall than what the plantation will aford onlly 6 gallons
of strong Drink."[11]

Another protest is voiced in the will of Captain George
Jordan, a leading planter of Surry County, in 1677: he re-
quests that he be buried in "Major Browne his Orchard, &
that at my buriall there may be no Drunckeness nor Gunns,
but a good and decent funerall to Entertaine my ffriends &
Neighbors. . . ."[12]

On the other hand Mrs. Alice Parke not only gave her
husband a fine funeral, but apparently combined it with a
wedding, for she demands 600 pounds of tobacco from the
court to reimburse her for the following expenses on behalf
of her deceased husband:

"p 2 fatt Calves, 1 Mutton, 12 dayes worke, 1 dayes worke
ffor a Butcher, 1 day to dress victualls, make grave, wed-
dinge & funerall charges, Box of pills & ffetchinge minister. . . ."[13]

---

[10]Henrico County Records, v. 1, p. 258.
[11]York County Records, v. 6, p. 484.
[12]Surry County Records, v. 2, p. 191.
[13]Ibid., v. 1, p. 113.

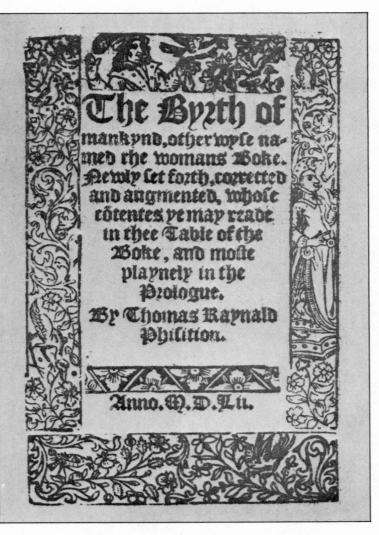

Title page of Raynald's *Birth of Mankind,* often found in Seventeenth Century Virginia libraries.

Nursing was at that time indeed a task for men, entailing physical labor that would horrify the modern nurse. Some of the women were apparently relieved by their husbands of the responsibility of collecting their bills. The records of Surry County in 1663 show that Ralph Creed presented a bill for his wife's attendance on a patient "with the comfortablest things a Man in his Condition could expect" and for the "entertainment of those that came to bury him wth 3 vollys of shott & diging his grave wth the trouble of his funeral included."[14] The estate of Captain Robert Spenser lists among its debts: "to pd. Mr. Plaw for his wife's tending Capt. Spenser . . . 350" (pounds of tobacco).[15] Ralph Langley left one pound sterling to the "good woman who shall dress me and put me in my coffin."[16]

It appears that at times the doctors' wives acted as nurses. Sarah Overstreete, a physician's widow, filed a bill in York County court in 1672 for her "trouble and pains" about Thomas Kotton in his sickness, and also "for funeral charges."[17]

The duties of the Seventeenth Century nurse were not to take the temperature, record the pulse, give daily baths, or follow elaborate orders from physicians; but to prepare food, give the "draughts regularly," wash the linen, watch by the bedside, and when death came (as it usually appeared

---

[14]Surry County Records, v. 1, p. 231.
[15]Ibid., v. 3, p. 79.
[16]York County Records, v. 6, p. 484.
[17]Ibid., v. 5, p. 321.

to do when the patient was ill enough to warrant a nurse) to shroud the body and to furnish the entertainment of those who came to the funeral.

II

Midwifery

Obstetrics was not a man's profession in America until the middle of the next century. John Moultrie, of Charleston, was the first regular obstetrician in this country. He died in 1775. The first lectures on midwifery were given by Shippen in 1765. Before this midwives were women, whose training was acquired in a crude apprenticeship or through unaided personal experience. Until the knowledge of antisepsis and the causes of puerperal sepsis were known, the midwife was perhaps safer than the obstetrician. The overzealous physician was apt to examine his patient before delivery and thus introduce an infection which would not have occurred if he had just waited, as did the women.[18]

Midwives played as important a part in other colonies as in Virginia. In New York they enjoyed unusual prestige and received rather liberal pay. At first the Dutch West India Company paid them. In 1655 Hellegond Jones was paid one hundred guilders by the Council for her obstetrical work among the poor. Early in the Seventeenth Century New

---

[18]Dr. W. A. Plecker of the Virginia Bureau of Vital Statistics has demonstrated this in an analysis of available statistics for deaths from puerperal sepsis in the negro and white races before 1860. He was able to show a much higher mortality among the whites attended by doctors than among the negroes attended by midwives.

York passed an ordinance governing midwives which throws
light upon the abuses which may also have been prevalent
in Virginia. An oath was exacted before the authorities,
binding the midwife to treat the rich and the poor alike, its
wording seeming to show that midwives not infrequently
left poor patients in order to attend those who could afford
to pay them higher fees. The ordinance further provides
against fraud, making it unlawful to misrepresent a child's
father, to be party to a false delivery or to conceal births,
especially the births of bastards. Midwives were pledged
to expose infanticide, to summon other midwives in suspicious cases, and not to induce abortion or charge
exorbitantly.[19]

In New England there were famous early midwives.
Mrs. Dr. Sam Fuller and Mrs. Anne Hutchinson of Boston,
Ruth Barnaby and poor Margaret Jones linger as well
known names. The Seventeenth Century Virginia midwives,
if not so illustrious, were no less busy, for it was a time of
large families. John Thruston recorded in an old book in
1652 that his wife was delivered of a daughter "who was
Baptized ye next day & named Rachell by Mr. Joseph Brint
Mindister, Mres Haywood midwife, and Sister Redby
Gossp, being my 20th child."[20]

We do not know the names of many Virginia midwives in
this century, but in Surry County in 1685 there was "Goodwife Thorpe, Midwife," whose fee was one hundred pounds

[19]Walsh: History of Medicine in N. Y.. v. 1, p. 21.
[20]William and Mary Quarterly, v. 4, p. 26.

of tobacco.[21]   In Isle of Wight County there was Hannah Webb, who wrote William Arundale that "yor Sonn William is one or two and twenty yrse of Age Janry next, for I delivered yor wife of him in ye younger Wm. Carters House."[22]   Mrs. Richard Hill was delivered in 1676 in Dr. George Lee's house by two midwives, assisted by two nurses and other women.   Dr. Lee does not appear to have been present.[23]   Susanna Evans, "age 60 yeares or thereabt," and Elizabeth Tindall were midwives in York County, 1677-1684.[24]   The widow Hollins was paid twelve hens for obstetrical services in 1634.[25]   Dorothey Bullock swore in 1662 that her delivery of Ann Roberts of a bastard child was her first case.[26]

The records show not a few bastard births.   Moral obliquity of this nature was not readily hidden in the small communities of colonial Virginia.   The unfortunate woman, usually of the servant class, if not forced to wear the scarlet letter was commonly punished publicly with stripes or prolonged servitude.   Dr. Daniel Parke's servant, Elizabeth Holloway, in 1662 was ordered to receive ten stripes on her bare back for her misconduct, and a servant of William Townsend in 1672 had to serve him two years longer, besides receiving twenty-nine lashes, for a similar offense.[27]

---

[21]Surry County Records, v. 3, p. 83.
[22]Ibid., v. 2, p. 38.
[23]Ibid., v. 2, p. 108.
[24]York County Records, v. 6, pp. 52, 606.
[25]Stanard: Story of Virginia's First Century, p. 195.
[26]York County Records, v. 3, p. 434.
[27]Ibid., v. 3, p. 435; v. 6, p. 228.

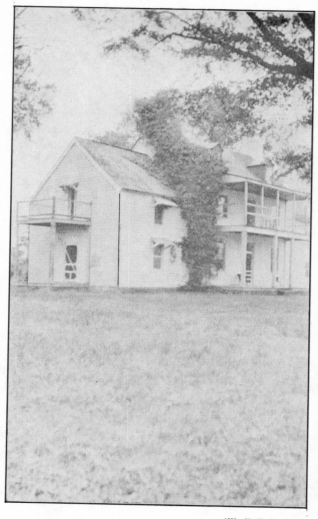

The house in which Grace Sherwood was tried for
witchcraft, still standing in Princess Anne County.

Midwives were called upon to serve on juries when the question of pregnancy was involved. Margaret Hatch, who was sentenced to be hanged in 1633 for murdering her child, pleaded pregnancy, but a "Jury of Matrons" found her "not pregnant."[28]

III

Witchcraft

There is a rather intimate association between medicine and witchcraft. The connection has not always done credit to the medical profession, as when Sir Thomas Browne assented to the deaths of the poor witches of Norwich. In New England the midwives, Ann Hutchinson and Margaret Jones, both won the stigma of witchcraft. In Virginia the Minutes of the Council and General Court for 1626 record a striking instance of how midwifery might lead to charges of witchcraft.

On September 11, 1626, testimony was given before the General Court concerning Goodwife Wright, who was accused of being a witch. Lieutenant Giles Allington testified that "he had spoken to good wiefe Wrighte for to bringe his wiefe to bed, but the saide good wief beinge left handed, his weife desired him to gett Mrs. Grave to be her midwiefe, wch this deponent did, and . . . the saide goodwiefe Wright went awaye from his howse very much discontented, in regarde the other midwiefe had brought his wiefe to bedd."

---

[28]Minutes of Council and General Court, Conway Robinson's notes for 1633.

Soon after this, his wife's breast "grew dangerouslie sore of an Imposture and was a moneth or 5 weeks before she was recovered, Att wch tyme This deponent him selfe fell sick and contynued the space of three weeks, And further sayeth yt his childe after it was borne fell sick . . . and so departed."

Rebecka Graye then testified that Goodwife Wright told her "yt she told Mr. ffellgate he should bury his wiefe (wch cam to pass) . . . and that she tolde Thomas Harris he should burie his first wiefe being then betrothed unto him (wch cam so to pass) . . ."

Several other witnesses told of Goodwife Wright's having prophesied deaths. Mrs. Pery swore "yt good wiefe Wright told her, that [when] she was at Hull her dame being sick suspected her selfe to be bewiched, and told good wiefe Wright of it, whereuppon by directione from her dame, That at the comeing of a woman, wch was suspected, to take a horshwe [horse-shoe] and flinge it into the oven and when it was red hott, To fflinge it into her dames urine, and so long as the horshwe was hott, the witch was sick at the harte, And when the Irone was colde she was well again, And this good wiefe Wright affirmeth to be trwe. . . ."[29]

The midwife might well be the ugly old woman popularly associated with witchcraft. Her superior knowledge and a certain mystery about her profession worked on the imagination of her neighbors. She was a sort of public character at

---

[29]Minutes of Council and General Court, pp. 111, 112.

a time when it was not wise for women to be too conspicuous.

Medicine touched witchcraft in another way. There were three infallible tests of a witch: 1. The presence in the suspect's house of "images," or "Pictures of Clay or Wax (like a Man, etc., made of such as they would bewitch) found in their House, or which they roast, or bury in the Earth, that as the Picture consumes, so may the parties bewitched consume." 2. The "water test," or ducking— "the pure water refusing to receive a witch into its bosom," guilt was established by failure to sink. 3. Witch marks— the witches being supposed to have "some big or little teat upon their body," which "being pricked will not bleed, and be often in their secretest parts, and therefore require diligent and careful search."[30] A jury of "ancient and knowing women" was required to settle this last point. They were usually the local midwives.

Still another medical ramification was the belief that the witch had power to cause sickness and death. This is illustrated in the case of Goodwife Wright, just quoted. In 1671 one Edward Cole was quoted as saying that "the suspition of Doctor Saunders & others was that his [Cole's] wife was under an ill tongue, & if it was soe he concluded yt it was Mrs. Neal by reason of imprecations made by her & yt indeed he thought soe, but since she came to his house and passed over the horseshoe nailed at ye door & prayed

---

[30]Burr: Narratives of the Witchcraft Cases, p. 440.

soe heartily for his wive's recovery, that suspition was gone
from him. . . ."[31]

Shortly before 1676 Colonel Mason captured the son of
the King of the Doegs and carried him home, after which
the boy lay in bed for ten days, his eyes staring and his
mouth agape, but with no sign that he was breathing, although his body was warm. Captain Brent, a Catholic,
examined him, said he was bewitched, and advocated bap-
tism. The boy was baptised and soon recovered.[32]

The hanging of Kate Grady at sea in 1658 is the only case
of the death of a witch which ever came into the Virginia
Courts.[33] William Harding was convicted of witchcraft in
1656 by an able jury of twenty-four men. The Northumberland County court ordered that he receive ten stripes
upon his bare back and be forever banished from the
County, two months being allowed him in which to collect
his belongings and depart.[34]

The traveler is still shown in Princess Anne County the
house in which Grace Sherwood was imprisoned. The
memorable witchcraft case, in which Grace was the defendant, is graphically recorded in the annals of the court:

"Whereas on complaint of Luke Hill on behalf of her
Majesty yt now is agt Grace Sherwood for prson Suspected
of witchcraft & having had Sundry Evdences Sworne agt

[31]Northumberland County Records, in William and Mary Quarterly,
v. 17, p. 248.
[32]Northampton County Records, v. 1657-64, p. 18.
[33]Lower Norfolk County Antiquary, v. 3, p. 52.
[34]William and Mary Quarterly, v. 1, p. 69.

her proving Many Cercumstances to which she could not make any excuse or Little or nothing to say in her own Behalf only Seemed to Rely on wt ye Court should Doe and there upon consented to be tryed in ye water & likewise to be Serched againe wch experiants being tryed & she Swiming wn therein & bound contrary To custom & ye Judgt of all ye spectators & afterwards being Serched by ffive antient weomen who have all Declared on Oath yt She is not like ym nor noe other woman yt they knew of having two things like titts on her private parts of a Black Coller being Blacker yn ye Rest of her Body all wch cercumstances ye Court weighing in their Consideracon Doe therefore ordr yt ye Sherr take ye Sd Grace Into his Costody & to Commit her body to ye Common Goal of this county there to Secure her by irons or otherwise Directed in ordr for her coming to ye Common Goale of ye county to bee brought to a ffuture Tryall there."[35]

The ducking took place on July 10, 1706, at a point of land on Lynnhaven Bay ever since known as "Witch Duck." After the water test Grace was again confined to jail until a future trial. Apparently the case was not prosecuted any further, for the next mention of her occurs thirty-four years later when the record shows her three sons presenting themselves in court to prove her will.[36]

On the whole, although a belief in witchcraft was widespread and cases involving supposed witches are fairly

---

[35]William and Mary Quarterly, v. 4, p. 18.
[36]Burr: Narratives of the Witchcraft Cases, p. 442.

numerous in the Virginia records, the courts were usually able to prevent extreme measures. An order of the Lower Norfolk County court provides that, "Whereas divrs dangerous & scandalous speeches have been raised by some psons concerning sevrall women in this Countie, termeing them to be Witches, whereby theire reputacons have been much impaired and their lives brought in question. . . . . It is by this Cort ordered that what pson soever shall hereafter raise any such like scandall, concerninge any partie whatsor, and shall not be able to pve the same, both upon oath, and by sufficient witness, such pson soe offending shall in the first place paie a thousand pounds of tob: and likewise be lyable to further Censure of the Cort."[37] The court, while demonstrating its own belief in the possibility of witchcraft, at least sees to it that the charge is not made maliciously. There are several cases where this and similar court orders are enforced and punishment duly inflicted upon those who had brought groundless accusations of witchcraft.

IV

Doctresses

Among the Indians there were instances of unusual medical knowledge being attributed to old women. In the Eighteenth Century there was an account of an old negro woman who was spoken of as a doctor, and this was probably true

---

[37]William and Mary Quarterly, v. 2, p. 58.

of some white women as well. Under the primitive conditions existing in the early years in Virginia, doctors' widows occasionally dispensed medical advice. As late as 1700 we find Mrs. Mary Seal, former wife of Dr. Power, winning a suit for four pounds seven shillings "for phisicall means, etc., by her administered in the time of Richard Dunbar's sickness."[38] In Henrico County in 1678 there is a deposition that "Benjamin Hatcher sent for ye wife of Edward Good he haveing a sore on his head desired this woman to know what she would have to cure it, she made answere she would refer it to him, he said if she . . . pformed a cure he would give honest satisfaction."[39]

Reverend John Clayton, writing to the Royal Society in 1688 of his observations in Virginia, reports that "A Gentlewoman, that was a notable female Doctress, told me, that a Neighbour being bit by a Rattle-Snake swelled excessively; some Days afterwards she was sent for, who found him swelled beyond what she thought it had been possible for a skin to contain, and very thirsty. She gave him oriental Bezoar shaved, with a strong Decoction of the aforesaid Dittany, whereby she recovered the Person."[40]

In 1678 a deposition shows that Richard Wyther, whose eyes were injured in a fight, "spent much time in getting medicines from Mrs. Grendons and others. . . ."[41]

---

[38]York County Records, v. 12, p. 314.
[39]Henrico County Records, v. 1, p. 79.
[40]Force: Tracts, v. 3, Letter from Mr. John Clayton, p. 44.
[41]Henrico County Records, v. 2, p. 57.

The inventory of Thomas Owen's estate in 1688 includes a debt "To Mrs Martha Stratton for trouble & means when ye decedt was lame & sick & unable to help himself ... 300 lb. tob."[42]

A glimpse is had in the Richmond County records of another "doctress," Catherine Shrewsbury, who evidently combined school teaching with medicine. Judgment was granted her in 1693 against Richard Tompkins for 300 pounds of tobacco for eighteen months schooling of his son. Later it is recorded that "the action brought by Catherine Shrewsbury vs. Peter Foxon for cure of his sore Legg" is dismissed, "the Deft [defendant] making Oath that the said Catherine had effected no such cure upon him."[43]

In spite of these beginnings the modern Trotulla had to wait a long time for recognition in Virginia. It was 1910 before woman physicians were admitted to membership in the Richmond Academy of Medicine.

---

[42]Henrico County Records, v. 2, p. 321.
[43]Richmond County Records, v. 1692-94, part 2, pp. 79, 80.

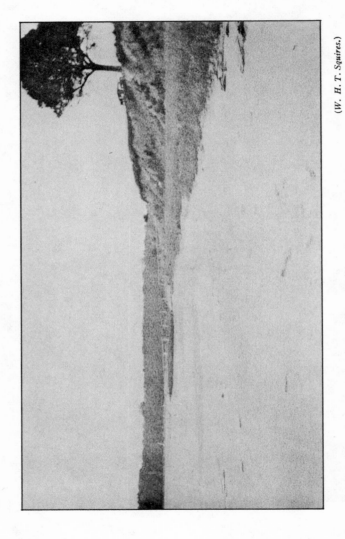

(*W. H. T. Squires.*)

Witch Duck, on Lynnhaven Bay, where Grace Sherwood underwent the ordeal by water.

CHAPTER VIII

THE PRIVATE LIFE OF PHYSICIANS

I

Houses

THE first houses at Jamestown were "built of rails and roofed with marsh grass thatch covered with earth." After the fire of 1608 they used boards for roofs and Indian mats on the walls. Floors were of dirt. Later, bark was used for the roof, "Wide and large country chimneys" were added, and clay was employed as plaster. Captain Smith left forty or fifty such houses in Jamestown in 1609. In 1611 there were some log houses with two stories and garret. In 1623 there were only twenty-two houses in Jamestown.[1] "For our howses & churches in those tymes they were so meane and poore by reason of those calamities that they could not stand above one or two yeeres."[2] Housebuilding in the capital was encouraged in 1636 by giving the builder his house, lot and garden plot.[3] In 1642 brickmaking was fostered in the colony by a grant of 500 acres for every house built of bricks. In 1661 the building of wooden homes was for-

[1]Virginia Magazine of History and Biography, v. 10, pp. 393-407.
[2]Journals of the House of Burgesses, v. 1619-1658/9, pp. 21, 22.
[3]Virginia Magazine of History and Biography, v. 10, pp. 393, 407.

bidden in Jamestown, and an abortive attempt was made to force each county to contribute a brick house to the capital.

Butler declared in his *Virginia Unmasked* that the houses were "the worst in the world" and that the most wretched cottages in England were superior to them. But this condition did not last long, and the increasing prosperity of the colony and the growing number of little land owners soon saw great improvement in the dwellings of the people. "Pleasant in their building," says John Hammond of the houses on the small plantations, "which although for most part they are but one story besides the loft, and built of wood, yet contrived so delightfully that your ordinary houses in England are not so handsome, for usually the rooms are large, daubed and whitelimed, glazed and flowered, and if not glazed windows, shutters which are made very pritty and convenient."[4] According to the *New Description of Virginia,* published in 1649, "They have lime in abundance for their houses, store of bricks made, and House and Chimnies built of Brick, and some of Wood high and fair, covered with Shingell for Tyle."[5]

What must have been a typical small planter's house is described in the Surry County records. A carpenter by the name of Felton contracted to build the house on the "plantation of Berkeley" for 1,400 pounds of tobacco, "wth a shedd

---

[4]Wertenbaker: Planters of Colonial Virginia, p. 104.
[5]Ibid.

all along the side, and a shedd at one End, wth a Chimney at the Inside at one End, and at the other End a Chimney without, and a Chimney at the side of the house on the outside. To partition the house into three Roomes and to lay the loft, and alsoe to build a Porch six foote wide and tenn foote longe. The timber to be brought in place, and the sd ffelton to Rive, Dubb, and Draw all boards . . . and the sd John Holmwood shall finde the sd ffelton suffit Diett while he is doing the sd worke."[6]

Some of the houses were more pretentious. That of Mrs. Elizabeth Diggs in 1692 contained, according to her inventory: "The Hall Parler, the Low Passage, the Yellow Room, the Large Roome against ye Yellow Room, Ye Back room agt ye large roome, Ye Red Room, Ye Garrett, and ye back Roome," in addition to servants' quarters and kitchen outside.[7] Katharine Thorpe's house in 1695 contained "Parlor, parlor chamber, chamber over ye parlor, Kitching, Hall, Hall Chamber."[8] The house of Nathaniel Bacon, the elder, included "ye Hall, ye inner Roome over ye Hall, Outer Roome, Madam Bacons Chamber, ye old Hall, ye chamber over ye old Hall, ye Chamber over Maddam Bacons, ye Shedd, ye Kitching, ye milk house."[9] James Whaley's inventory listed, "Hall chamber, the Hall, the Chamber, the Parlor, the kitchen chamber, the chamber

[6]Surry County Records, v. 1, p. 18.
[7]York County Records, v. 9, p. 215.
[8]Ibid., v. 11, p. 190.
[9]Ibid., v. 11, p. 261.

over ye parlor, the kitchen, the old store, the Seller, the entry, Mr. Whaley's closet."[10]

There are few descriptions of houses belonging to physicians, but from the size of their inventories and from their social status it is probable that most of them lived in small three or four-room cottages, of humble though comfortable proportions. Stephen Gill, who was a Captain and a Burgess as well as a physician, had a house with a "Hall, Chamber & inner Chamber, Shedd, Kitchen, Milk house."[11] Dr. Giles Modé's house consisted of a hall, chamber, little room, new room, cellar and kitchen.[12] Dr. Francis Haddon's inventory mentions "Chamber above stairs, Lower chamber, Hall, Stoare."[13]

II

Furniture

The inventories and wills of physicians, found in the Seventeenth Century county records, illumine a corner of their private life that is not without its surprises. The lists of household goods give a vivid picture of the poverty of those days. Physicians were probably richer than the average citizen, yet there is not the least indication of luxury and little of bare comfort in the carefully detailed catalogues of their evidently cherished possessions. A few specimens speak for themselves.

---

[10]York County Records, v. 12, p. 412.
[11]Ibid., v. 1, p. 56.
[12]Ibid., v. 2, p. 58.
[13]Ibid., v. 5, p. 196-198.

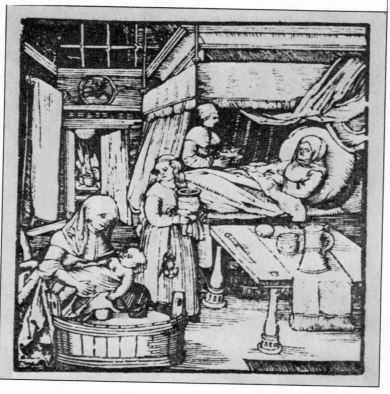

Obstetrical scene, from Raynald's *Birth of Mankind*, a book often found in Seventeenth Century Virginia libraries.

Nathaniel Knight, who died in Surry County in 1678, left "1 old feather bed & bolster, 1 sea bed, 2 trading cloth Blanket 1 old coverlet . . . 3 old Sadless & bridles: 1 old razor & hone, 2 glas dram cups, 2 horne ditto, 1 combe Case with a glass in it, 2 hornes with some powder . . . 1 small old Chest, 1 small old trunk, 1 gall glass bottle, 2 wine glasses, . . . 1 Semetar & belt, 1 pistall, 1 small gunn, A pcell of old bookes & some trifles besides . . ." in addition to his wearing apparel—the whole valued at 1,910 pounds of tobacco.[14]

Dr. John Severne's inventory, appraised in Northampton County in 1644 and valued at 2,847 pounds of tobacco, consisted of a few pewter and brass dishes, 2 old bedsteads, several sheets, one chair, 3 old chests, 2 feather beds, one parcel of old books, 5 geese and ganders, 1 pair of brass scales, 1 pair gold weights and a few other household articles.[15]

Dr. Giles Modé's furniture in 1657 included six leather chairs, several feather beds, cupboard, chest, 1 looking glass, a couch, 2 tables, sheets, towels and napkins.[16]

Dr. Isaac Clopton's will was probated in 1678. He bequeathed to his wife a tract of land, several men servants, feather beds, pewter dishes, sheets, towels, cows and wearing apparel.[17]

---

[14]Surry County Records, v. 2, p. 168-169.
[15]Northampton County Records, v. 1640-45, p. 338.
[16]York County Records, v. 2, p. 58.
[17]Ibid., v. 6, p. 133.

Dr. Peter Plovier's will in 1677 disposed of a feather bed and a heifer.[18]   He also owned some tracts of land.

Dr. Henry Power in 1693 left 5 feather beds (one of them, with its "furniture," valued at 7 lb. 10 s.), "6 lethern chaires," "one houre glass," cupboards, chests, trunks, chest of drawers, 2 silk pincushions, 7 table cloths, 39 napkins, 16 pewter dishes, 2 plates, 18 spoons, a Tumbler, 3 cups, a quart pott, a powdering tubb, a powder horn, a tinder box, 10 "pillow bears," 6 towels, and "3 servants with their beds."[19]

Dr. John Holloway in 1643 left an estate larger than the average.   It included 2 chairs, 6 stools, 2 feather beds, 6 flock beds, sheets (some Holland and some canvas), a looking glass, 2 swords & daggers, 5 guns, 1 pistoll, 8 candle-sticks, pewter porringers, dishes and spoons, 61 cattle, 16 goats, 22 poultry and "The Plantacon, Cropp corne & Tobacco," besides his wearing apparel.[20]

Most of these inventories are taken from the last half of the century, as there are few of the earlier ones remaining. They represent, therefore, the improved living conditions that followed a generation of settlement.   The furniture of the earlier log cabin period must have been even simpler. In the first half of the century stools and benches usually took the place of chairs.   When chairs became more common, they were ponderous affairs of carved oak, the so-

---

[18]York County Records, v. 6, p. 50.
[19]Ibid., v. 9, p. 293.
[20]Northampton County Records, v. 1640-45, pp. 257-259.

called wainscot chairs. Upholstery was used, some of it "turkey worked." Later there were wicker chairs, Russia leather chairs, willow chairs, but no mahogany until after 1740. Feather beds were highly valued. Flock beds, stuffed with rags and cotton, were often used instead. Bedsteads were huge and high, with a trundle bed underneath for the children. Chests, plain or carved, corner cupboards and tables, usually very plain, completed the furniture of the period. An article often mentioned was the lookingglass. There were sheets, towels, napkins, pillow biers, pewter porringers, dishes and spoons, and an occasional rug. The absence of certain articles is notable. There are no clocks, few watches, no lamps, pictures, rocking chairs, knives, forks or china, and very little glass.

III

Dress

Standing before the wax effigies in Westminster Abbey, one cannot help feeling something of the personality which the now faded splendor of their dress once clothed. So a glimpse into the wardrobes of early Virginia physicians rewards us with a genuine sense of their reality.[21]

Captain John Smith advised the adventurer to Virginia to outfit himself with a Monmouth cap, 3 falling bands, 3 shirts, 1 waist coat, 1 suit of canvas, 1 of frieze, 1 of

---

[21]Earle: *Two Centuries of Costume in America* contains a valuable account of the dress of the Seventeenth Century American, and is used in some of the descriptions in this section.

broadcloth, 3 pair stockings, 4 pair shoes and a dozen points. Sword, gun and armor were recommended as useful.[22]

Dr. Bohun was probably a familiar figure on the streets of Jamestown in 1610. He wore knee breeches, stockings and the heavy shoes of the day. A tight fitting doublet covered his Holland shirt. A ruff, made up of yards of plaited linen, may have adorned his neck, though it is hard to think of starch and pinking irons in a wilderness. A Monmouth cap covered his short hair, and his beard grew unshaven as it did on all men of that day.

As the century wore on, head dresses changed completely. Perukes and periwigs made their appearance, and long powdered curls hung to the shoulders. They must have been exceedingly hot and disagreeable, certainly they were heavy, expensive and dirty. With the advent of the wig the beard went into the discard. Likewise went the ruffs and the falling bands. Our Virginia doctor now appears quite changed. Into his periwig he has just dusted two pounds of powder, which is stuck there by a nauseous glue. He is clean shaven and wears cravat, vest, knee breeches, garters and buckles. His coat reaches to the knees and may or may not be ornamented with embroidery. He wears the Cavalier or the steeple-crowned hat. When his day is done he goes to rest in his impressive feather bed, and should he be disturbed by a night call he will appear at the window in night cap and rails. If he is less well to do, he sleeps in a

---

[22]Smith: General History of Virginia, p. 607.

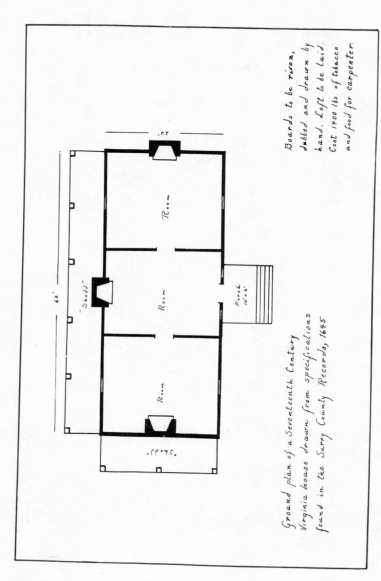

Ground plan of a Seventeenth Century Virginia house.

flock bed, in day shirt or nude, in an apartment shared by
his family and sometimes by strangers.

Looking into the inventories of the physician, we see what
he actually left.   Dr. Holloway's wearing apparel included
2 waistcoats, stockings, caps, shirts, 2 pair shoes, several
pair drawers, a cloak, and "ffringed gloves."   This was in
1643.[23]   Andrew Winter in 1679 left a "doublet, coat,
breaches black and a hatt," valued at 300 pounds of tobacco;
"foure worne shirts, six pairs of old worn Drawers one pair
old thread stockings," worth 150 pounds of tobacco; and
"foure old neckclothes, two pair cuffs and seven bands,"
estimated at 300 pounds of tobacco.   He also had a cane
and a pair of cordovan gloves.[24]   Nathaniel Knight in 1678
left personal effects as follows:

> "2 Dimity wastcots
> 1 p Drawers
> 1 very old holland shirt
> 1 half ditto
> 1 p old holland drawers
> 1 cravatt
> 3 p old holland Sleeves and Ruffles
> 8 old holland bands
> 1 p old gloves
> 1 caster hat
> 2 small black felts
> 1 old Kersey Coate
> 1 new Kersey ditto

[23]Northampton County Records, v. 1640-45, pp. 257-259.
[24]York County Records, v. 6, p. 171.

2 p briches
3 cotton wast coats & Drawers."[25]

Clothes were expensive and scarce. Physicians sometimes took old clothes in settlement of an account, and a legacy of old clothes was worth receiving. When Chirurgeon John Stringer treated Richard and Edward Newport for the plague (of which both patients died), it was "thought requisite and accordingly ordered by this Cort That . . . hee shall have the weareing apparell that hee is now possessed of that did then belong to the sd Newport and one hogd of tobacco. . . ."[26] In 1685 Michael Sherlock, of Rappahannock County, petitioned the court for the wearing apparel left him by the will of Dr. Roger Water.[27] From the estate of John Vaden Dr. Symonds received in 1679 "500 lb of tob & 2 paire of french falls."[28] The effects of Robert Austin contained in 1626 "some old clothes & a hatt," which he had given "to such as tended him in his sickness."[29]

IV

Wives

Women were important factors in the colony's life. Not only were they nurses, midwives and doctresses, but as wives of doctors they must feed and house their husbands' ap-

---

[25]Surry County Records, v. 2, p. 169.
[26]Northampton County Records. 1640-45, pp. 218, 219.
[27]Rappahannock County Records, v. 10, p. 117.
[28]York County Records, v. 6, p. 157.
[29]Minutes of Council and General Court, in Virginia Magazine of History and Biography, v. 27, p. 35.

prentices as well as the patients so often cared for in the physician's own home.   In addition these stout frontier women seem to have found time to learn a little medicine on the side, and one of them, Mrs. Pott, braved the long voyage to England to plead for her husband's pardon.

Remarriages were common, and Virginia widows contracted new alliances with great speed.   Colonel Byrd declared that marriage thrived exceedingly and that an old maid or an old bachelor was as scarce and "as ominous as a Blazing star."   Mrs. Dr. Modé became Mrs. Dr. Haddon after less than four months of widowhood.   Dr. Holloway's widow was likewise without a husband for a bare four months.   Mrs. Peter Plovier's second husband probated the will of her first, and Mrs. Henry Power had already married Mr. Seal when she presented to the court the inventory of Dr. Power's estate.

V

Transportation

In the early days when the settlements were chiefly along the waterways and roads were poor, the common means of transportation was by boat.   In 1660 Samuel Strachey was fined 350 pounds of tobacco for borrowing Dr. Patrick Napier's boat, because of "the great priudice done ye said Napier for want of ye same being yen visiting his sick patients & forced to wayt for his boat a long time."[30]   As late as 1680 the debts of Henrico County included: "To

---

[30]York County Records, v. 3, p. 204.

Henry Jordan for 25 days rowing Burgesses . . . 275"
(pounds of tobacco).[31]

Inland travel came slowly. In 1632 (about the time the
counties were created) it was decreed that "Highwayes
shall be layd out in such convenient places as are requisite."[32]
In 1657 a statute provided that "surveyors of highwayes
and maintenance for bridges be yearly kept & appointed in
each countie court . . . respect being had to the course used
in England to that end."[33] In Henrico County in 1683 the
county surveyors are ordered to "cause ye sd ways to be
cleared forty feet wide, and bridle Roads to all houses according to law."[34] The Virginia law prescribed in 1694
that "Justices yearly in October Court appoint such who
shall lay out convt waies to church, Court, Jamestown and
from County to County 40 foot broad and bridges where
Occasion."[35] Still the highways were often neglected and
impassable. Late in the century we find orders directing
that the roads be cleared "to be passable & safe for man
and horse to travell without danger of damage," and again,
"so that horse and poste may be safe." Complaint was
raised in 1693 because "the wayes not cleared for two
years space from Mount My Ladyes up to ye falls."[36] The
surveyors of Surry County were indicted in 1675 by the
Grand Jury "for yr neglect."

31Henrico County Records, v. 1, p. 146.
32Hening: Statutes at Large, v. 1, p. 199.
33Ibid., v. 1, p. 436.
34Henrico County Records, v. 2, p. 145.
35Virginia Magazine of History and Biography, v. 10, p. 53.
36Henrico County Records, v. 5, p. 407.

The rough roads intimately concerned the physician. One associates the rural doctor with long hours of travel, day and night, plodding weary roads. His life and his comfort were peculiarly bound up with the condition of the highways. In spite of statutes providing for forty foot roadways many of the colonial roads were mere bridle paths, impassable for vehicles, especially in winter. There were, indeed, few vehicles in Virginia in this century. Major Peter Walker's inventory in 1656 was typical of many others. It included seven servants and three horses, but no vehicles. Among the numerous inventories of physicians' estates not a single instance of a vehicle has been found. Stephen Gill, Chirurgeon and Burgess of York County, in 1653 had seven servants but no vehicle, only "1 horse and saddle."[37] Nathaniel Hill in 1690 left "2 horses, saddles and bridles."[38] Dr. Giles Modé died in 1657, leaving an estate covering three pages of the record. He had seven horses, but not so much as a "jumper" to hitch them to.[39] The Swiss traveller, Michel, observed that horses were very common. "Going to church means at some places a trip of more than thirty miles, but . . . it is not a great hardship, because people are well mounted there. Horses, which are hardly used for anything else but riding, are half deers. They run always in a fast gallop. . . ."[40]

---

[37]York County Records, v. 1, pp. 56-58.
[38]Henrico County Records, v. 5, p. 182.
[39]York County Records, v. 2, p. 58.
[40]Virginia Magazine of History and Biography, v. 24, "Journey of Michel from Switzerland to Virginia."

VI

Outdoor Life

Early Virginians were fond of outdoor life. Francis Nicholson, who was Governor in 1690, attempted among his first acts to recoup the popularity he had lost in New York by introducing public sports. He established and proclaimed field days in all the counties. Horse racing, however, was the popular sport in Virginia as in England. The quarter mile was the favorite racing distance. An amusing early reference to the sport is found in the York County records for 1674, and concerns Dr. Matthew Slader:

"James Bullocke a Tayler having made a race for his mare to run with a horse belonging to Mr. Mathew Slader for two thousand pounds of tobaccoe & caske & it being contrary to lawe for a labourer to make a race being a sport only for gentlemen is fined for the same one hundred pounds of tobaccoe & caske.

"Whereas Mr Mathew Slader & James Bullocke by condicon under hand & seale made a race for two thousand pounds of tabaccoe & caske & it appearing under the hand & seale of the said Slader that his horse should runn out of the way that Bullocke's mare might winn wch is an apparent cheate is orded to be putt in the stocks & there to sitt the space of an houre."[41]

---

[41]York County Records, v. 5, p. 167.

Rum was often mixed with horse racing, for drinking seems to have been common enough. There were twenty indictments for drunkenness at one sitting of a Henrico County Grand Jury in 1678.[42] At a time when china and glass were rare the effects of Nathaniel Knight contained two wine glasses and two glass dram cups. Dr. Francis Taylor swore in Surry County court in 1674 that he bought his ale, beer and rum from Walter Bartlett.[43] Other evidence that Virginia doctors took part in the general convivial life of the colony is furnished by Thomas Gerard, a well known physician of Westmoreland County, who in 1670 was associated with John Lee, Henry Corbin and Isaac Allerton in building a "banqueting house" on their adjoining land.[44]

VII

Morals

The Church of England had a firm hand on the religious life of the colony, though the Virginia of this century was not noted for its piety. The doctors of the period do not appear prominently in church affairs. Richard Dunning, "ch. warden of New Pawquoson p'ish,"[45] and Walter Whitaker, vestryman of Christ Church,[46] are the only physicians we have found serving on vestries before 1700. Sunday observance and church going were matters of law.

---

[42]Henrico County Records, v. 1, p. 70.
[43]Surry County Records, v. 2, p. 56.
[44]Neill: Virginia Carolorum, p. 255.
[45]York County Records, v. 2, p. 414.
[46]Christ Church, Middlesex County Vestry Book, p. 16.

In 1623 it cost five pounds of tobacco to absent oneself from church. In 1642 it was unlawful to make a journey on the Sabbath Day. Dr. Nathaniel Knight in 1675 was one of twenty-eight men presented to the Grand Jury for "not frequenting ye church."[47] In 1692 Dr. John Bowman was brought before the Grand Jury "for swearing 2 oaths."[48] The court of Northampton County in 1642 ordered that "John Holloway, Chir: shalbe amerc't. 30 lb. tob. for swearing a blasphemous oath in the face of the open court. . . ." The same Holloway four years earlier had been required to confess before the congregation that he had committed the "sin of fornication," and had been fined 200 pounds of tobacco. On another occasion, for failing to answer a summons, he was ordered to "lay neck and heels at the church dore one the next Sabbath Day."[49]

In 1655 Chirurgeon James Taylor's wife sued for a separation, swearing in her deposition that her husband "hath kept a Whore in the house ever since he married her" and that therefore she "desireth a sepparation and to goe live with her Mother and to have a considerable maintenance allowed her. . . ."[50]

Dr. Pott was convicted of cattle stealing, Dr. Slader cheated in a horse-race, and George Gunnell, an Elizabeth City County chirurgeon, was sought in 1689 for debts and

---

[47]Surry County Records, v. 2, p. 83.
[48]Henrico County Records, v. 5, p. 322.
[49]Northampton County Records, v. 1632-40, pp. 24, 123; v. 1640-45, p. 169.
[50]Surry County Records, v. 1, p. 40.

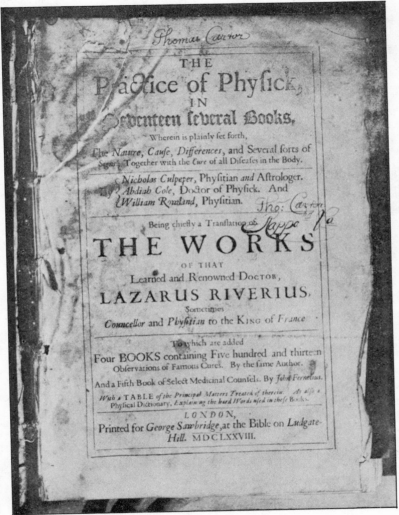

Thomas Carter

THE
Practice of Physick,
IN
Seventeen several Books,
Wherein is plainly set forth,
The Nature, Cause, Differences, and Several sorts of Signs; Together with the Cure of all Diseases in the Body.

Nicholas Culpeper, Physitian and Astrologer.
Abdiah Cole, Doctor of Physick. And
William Rowland, Physitian.

Being chiefly a Translation of

THE WORKS
OF THAT
Learned and Renowned Doctor,
LAZARUS RIVERIUS,
Sometimes
Councellor and Physitian to the King of France

To which are added
Four BOOKS containing Five hundred and thirteen Observations of Famous Cures. By the same Author.
And a Fifth Book of Select Medicinal Counsels. By John Fernelius.
With a TABLE of the Principal Matters Treated of therein. As also a Physical Dictionary, Explaining the hard Words used in these Books.

LONDON,
Printed for George Sawbridge, at the Bible on Ludgate-Hill. MDCLXXVIII.

(Library of the Richmond Academy of Medicine, Miller Collection.)

Title page of Riverius's *Practice of Physic,* a book often found in Seventeenth Century Virginia libraries.

"absconded himself" into Maryland.[51]   Physicians were not, however, the only sinners.   "Mr. Thomas Hampton, Cle" (minister) of York County, after obtaining the guardian-ship of the orphans of John Powell, was accused of ap-propriating their estates, taking one of the orphans and most of the estate out of the county, and leaving behind "the other orphant by name Wm Powell without necessary pr'vson to say even starke naked."[52]

It does not require great imagination to see our Seven-teenth Century doctor dressed in knee breeches and jerkin, perhaps adorned with periwig and cap; not given to church-going, but fond of ale, horse-racing and cuss words; husband of a multiparous wife; owner of a log cabin home or at best a frame cottage which he guarded with gun, pistol and scimitar; his road a bridle path and his means of conveyance a horse or boat.   We find him caring for his patients in his own house; tutoring apprentices; reading old Latin text books by candle light, without spectacles; writing with a goose quill pen; sitting on a rough stool or bench; eating at a crude table from pewter dishes, without fork or table knife; having no knowledge of bath tubs; keeping his clothes in trunk or chest; sleeping, night-capped, on a flock bed in a bedroom shared by others; dividing his time, which he measured with hour-glass and sundial, among medicine, politics and farming; often in court, often a justice, member of Council or Assembly, and subject, like his neighbors, to military service.

---

[51]Elizabeth City County Records, v. 1684-99, p. 293.
[52]York County Records, v. 2, p. 190.

CHAPTER IX

PUBLIC LIFE OF PHYSICIANS

I

Military Service

HE defense of the colony was entirely in the hands of the county militia, organized under the command of a County Lieutenant, who corresponded somewhat to the Lord Lieutenant of the English shires. Since a large portion of the population was subject to military service[1] and there was a corresponding number of officers, the colony seemed to be teeming with titled gentlemen. One observer remarked that "wherever you travel in Maryland (as also in Virginia and Carolina) your ears are astonished at the number of colonels, majors and captains that you hear mentioned."[2] Physicians in military service appear usually to have been called by their military titles only when serving as line officers.

Dr. Pott was a captain of musketeers. Dr. Daniel Parke rose from captain and major to colonel. Dr. John Stone was usually referred to as "Colonel Stone." Dr. Walter Whitaker was captain of militia in Middlesex, and Dr.

---

[1]Bruce states that the militia numbered 9,522 at the end of the century. Virginia Magazine of History and Biography, v. 24, p. 24.
[2]London Magazine, 1745.

Henry Whiting was a major of horse in the Gloucester militia. Other physicians who were not line officers played their part when the militia took the field. In 1644 an expedition against the Indians was planned in retaliation for the recent massacre, and among the orders of the General Assembly is one "that Mr. Henry Luellin bee entertayned as Chirurgeon Generall for the Armye to Pomunkey and to contynue in that Imployment, and to have pay at the Publique Charge. Allsoe that Doctor Waldron Mr Dunnington and Mountayne Rowland or some of them bee desired to goe along wth them."[3]   Act XIII of the Grand Assembly, March 21, 1645, provided "that the Leu'ts and dept. Leu'ts do take care to provide a sufficient chirurgeon for the said forte," namely Fort Henry, the site of the present city of Petersburg.[4]   Jonathan Grover was given a commission in 1676 as surgeon to the "five companies of foot guards employed by the king in an expedition to Virginia under command of Capt. Herbert Jeffrey."[5]   In 1680 an order of the Assembly mentions medicines delivered to Robert Synock, "Surgeon to Rappahannock Garison."[6]   John Julian, chirurgeon of the Potomac garrison in 1682, received "for twenty five daies, 764" pounds of tobacco.[7]   In 1679 the surgeon of a garrison received 850 pounds of tobacco a month.[8]

[3]Virginia Magazine of History and Biography, v. 23, p. 233.
[4]William and Mary Quarterly, v. 3, p. 5 (second series.)
[5]Calendar British State Papers, v. 1675-77, p. 460.
[6]Bruce: Institutional History of Virginia, v. 2, p. 108.
[7]Journals House of Burgesses, v. 1659-93, p. 173.
[8]Bruce: Institutional History of Virginia, v. 2, p. 14.

The military expedition, sent to Virginia from England in 1676 to put down the Indians and restore order after Bacon's Rebellion, called forth the following surgical provisions: "Memorandum concerning provisions and necessaries for sick men in Virginia calculated as is usual at 12d. per head for six months; . . . and likewise for setting apart money for the surgeon's chest, about 53 lb. That my Lord Treasurer take order for payment of the same upon account to John Knight, Surgeon-General."[9] About the same time it was provided that "the commander of each important division of the forces was authorized to impress two physicians to attend to the medical wants of his troops."[10] Eight forts were planned, to protect the settlements against Indian attacks which were rife at that time. They were to extend from the Potomac to the Nansemond, about forty miles intervening between each fort. The General Assembly voted that each of the eight forts was to be supplied with a chirurgeon, furnished with "a convenient supply of medicines & salves, etc. to the value of five pounds sterling for every hundred men. . . ."[11]

In the early years of the century the military commander of each hundred acted as the chief commisioner of health for his district. Later a commander was appointed for each county.[12] Physicians were not exempt from military duty until May 1691, when an exception was made in their favor,

[9]Calendar British State Papers, v. 1675-76, p. 484.
[10]Bruce: Institutional History of Virginia, v. 2, p. 88.
[11]William and Mary Quarterly, second series, v. 3, p. 7.
[12]Bruce: Institutional History of Virginia, v. 2, p. 17.

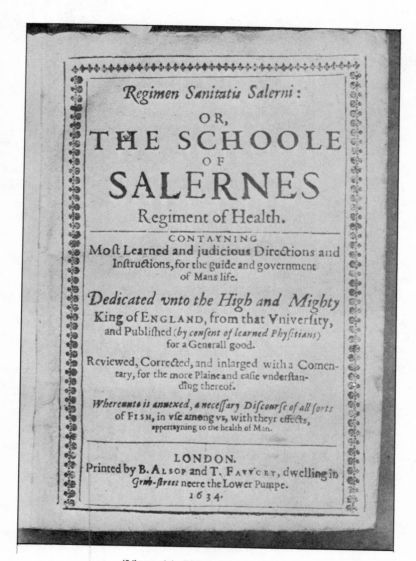

Regimen Sanitatis Salerni :

OR,

THE SCHOOLE

OF

SALERNES

Regiment of Health.

CONTAYNING

Most Learned and judicious Directions and
Instructions, for the guide and government
of Mans life.

Dedicated vnto the High and Mighty
King of ENGLAND, from that Vniversity,
and Published *(by consent of learned Physitians)*
for a Generall good.

Reviewed, Corrected, and inlarged with a Comen-
tary, for the more Plaine and easie vnderstan-
ding thereof.

Whereunto is annexed, a necessary Discourse of all sorts
of FISH, in vse among vs, with theyr effects,
appertayning to the health of Man.

LONDON.

Printed by B. ALSOP and T. FAVVCET, dwelling in
Grub-street neere the Lower Pumpe.
1 6 3 4.

Title page of the *Regimen Sanitatis,* a book often found in
Seventeenth Century Virginia libraries.

the Council ordering the militia officers not to enlist "Physicians Chirurgeons Readers Clerks Ferrymen Negroes."[13]

II

Office Holders

If military duty took some physicians away from their strictly professional pursuits, office-holding appears to have engaged a far greater number. Physicians seem to have held every position from Governor down. John Pott was Governor in 1629. He had also been in the Council. Other physician members of the Council were Richard Townshend, 1642, Obedience Robins, 1655, and Henry Whiting, 1691. Whiting had been Treasurer as well, and Daniel Parke also held both positions, as well as that of Secretary of State.[14]

Physicians in the House of Burgesses were Obedience Robins, Northampton, 1629-52; Richard Townshend, Charles River, 1641-42; Henry Poole, Elizabeth City, 1647-48; Henry Lee, Northumberland, 1651-52; Stephen Gill, York, 1652; Robert Ellyson, James City, 1655-56, 1663; John Stringer, Northampton, 1658-59; Daniel Parke, York, 1666; Robert Williamson, Isle of Wight, 1663, 1666.[15] Thomas Gerard, of Westmoreland County, had been a Privy Councillor of Maryland.[16]

---

[13]Executive Journals, Council of Colonial Virginia, v. 1, p. 526.
[14]Virginia Magazine of History and Biography, v. 9, p. 173; v. 18, p. 357; v. 14, p. 174.
[15]Journals House of Burgesses, v. 1619-1658/59; Virginia Magazine of History and Biography, v. 28, p. 326.
[16]Neill: Virginia Carolorum, p. 255.

The position of High Sheriff was sought after and held by a number of physicians, among them Robert Ellyson, Walter Whitaker, Richard Parker, Daniel Parke, William Bankes, Thomas Iken and John Stone. Stone, Parke and Whitaker had each been Justice of the Peace, as had Henry Lee, Henry Whiting, Richard Townshend, John Hay, Giles Modé and Isaac Clopton.

Physicians who served as appraisers and administrators of estates were William Irby, Henrico, 1695; George Eland, Elizabeth City; Walter Whitaker, of Middlesex; Thomas Culmer, of Surry, 1662; Moses Hubbart, Rappahannock, 1685; John Stringer, Northampton, 1643; and Godfrey Spruell, Henrico, 1690. Many doctors served at inquests and on coroner's juries. In such a capacity we encounter George Eland, 1695, John Stringer, 1642, John Peteet, 1659, Jeremiah Rawlins, 1661, Jeoffrey Wilson, 1659, Robert Ellyson, 1657, and John Overstreet, 1657.

III

Coroners

The office of coroner is a very ancient one. In England the duties formerly included caring for the interests of the Crown, especially where crown property was involved, as in shipwrecks, in judgments of outlawry and in cases of deodands. The coroner, of course, also passed on sudden and suspicious deaths. In England the coroners at first were none but "lawful and discreet knights," who served without pay. Fees were allowed in the time of Henry VII, but the mercenary character the office then assumed was deprecated by both Coke and Blackstone. Among the positions brought over bodily from the mother country by the colonists was that of coroner. Here he was at first a man of much importance, and some of the most distinguished Virginians held the office. Among them were William Randolph, William Byrd, the elder, John Farrar, Thomas and Richard Cocke, and James Minge.[17] Coroners were not necessarily physicians until 1910. At least two coroners were appointed annually in each parish by the Governor.[18] The coroner's jury consisted of six jurors who were required "to inquire, upon the view of the body of . . . there lying dead, when, how and by what means he came to his death." In Seventeenth Century Virginia a chirurgeon was usually a member of the jury.

The duties of the coroner in Virginia were multiple. He held inquests in cases of suspicious death. At times he was required to return "an account of all waifes strays and Deodands" within his county. Occasionally he had to act as administrator of the deceased's estate. At a General Court at James City, April 1687, "Mr. William Sherwood Corroner of James Citty County humbly begg'd leave of his Excellency & ye rest of ye Justices Sitting in Court to mind them, that according to Act of Parliament all Corroners are bound to p'sent to ye next assize all Inquisicions of ye death

---

[17]Henrico County Records, v. 1.
[18]Fiske: Old Virginia and her Neighbors, v. 2, p. 39.

of men by misfortune, violence or willful act, & conceiving ye Genll Court to be in ye nature of an Assize did humbly begg leave to offer to ye Courts consideracon whether it was not fitt & necessary that all Inquisitions by ye Corroner taken . . . be returned to ye Secretaryes office every Genll Court there to be Registered. . . ." The Court replied that this should be done "the Sixth day of each Genll Court, and that ye Same be duely Registered by ye Clk of ye office in book appointed for that use, and that ye fee for ye same be thirty pds of tobacco to be paid in like manner as ye Corroners fee is. . . . And whereas Several Horses and other Beasts doth stray at some distance . . . from ye grounds . . . of ye owners & are too often privately . . . kept by psons who have noe Right unto them. . . . The Court . . . direct that whoever takes up any stray horse or other beast shall give notice to ye Corroner of ye County . . . to ye intent ye Corroner may give publiq notice thereof by a note Sett up ye third day of every Genll Court. . . ." Such beasts, if unclaimed within twelve months, were to be sold by the coroner, the proceeds going to the auditor for His Majesty's use.[19]

Many of the inquests recorded in the Virginia County courts are full of interest. In 1653 a Surry County jury was ordered to inquire into the cause of the death of John Briant, "whither . . . by ye hand of men, or by the Kick or tread of a horse, or by a ffall agt a stump or tree, or by the Infirmity of any disease . . . . If by the hand of man, then

---

[19]Henrico County Records, v. 1, p. 453.

wth wt weapon. . . . And whither ye wounds or blows of
ye sd weapon were ye imeadiate cause of death or not. . . ."
The verdict was that he died of natural causes.[20]

In 1662 another jury finds that "William Billings by being
a servant who had beene not long before very sick in the
distemper vulgerly called Seasoninge, & being not well Recovered: was growne weak & was sent into the woods to
keepe Cattell: being ill at ease & Inclyninge to a Carelesse
dispare: did not soe carefully Indeavor his owne preservation as a healthy full & contented person would have done,
but . . . remaininge in the wood night & day . . . that hee con-
tinueinge without ffoode or other suckour in the woods hee
remained so untill hee became a dead corps. . . ."[21]

In 1675 a jury reports that a runaway maid servant died
"by reason of a distemper called the Scurvy."[22] A coroner's
jury in York County in 1660 examines a corpse and reports
that "finding his body free from bruises & wounds suppose
hee dyed of a surfeit. . . ."[23]

The ordeal of touch—stroking the corpse, as it was
called—was apparently a common resort of justice in the
Seventeenth Century.[24] Over it presided the coroner.
There is a mediaeval flavor to such accounts as that found
in the Accomac records for 1680. In a case of infanticide

---

[20]Surry County Records, v. 1, p. 31.
[21]Ibid., v. 1, p. 199.
[22]Ibid., v. 2, p. 95.
[23]York County Records, v. 3, p. 235.
[24]The theory was that if the person who stroked the corpse was guilty
of murder the corpse would move or show some alteration.

the coroner and a jury of twelve women reported that they
had "caused to be taken out of the ground in the garden"
the body of the "dead bastard child," and "then we caused
Sarah the wife of Paul Carter . . . to touch, handle and
stroake ye childe, in wch time we saw no alteration in the
body of ye childe; afterwards we called for Paul Carter
to touch ye s'd child and immediately while he was strook-
ing ye childe the black and sotted places about the body of
the childe grew fresh and red so that blud was redy to come
through ye skin of the child. We also observed the countenance of the said Paul Carter to alter into very much pale-
ness. . . ." As a result of this and other evidence the regular jury indicted Sarah and Paul for murder.[25]

In Northampton County the jury reported at an inquest
in 1656 that they "have viewed the body of Paul Rynnuse
late of this county dec[d] & have caused Mr. Wm. Custis to
touch the face & stroke the body of the said Paul Rynure
(which he very willingly did.) But no sign did appear unto
us of question in the law."[26]

Inquiring into the death of a maid servant of Peter Green,
a coroner's jury in 1662 reported that they "caused the said
Green and his wife to touch the Corps, And cannot find any
signs or tokens of any blows or kicks . . . and to our Judgments shee dyed naturally. . . ."[27]

In 1664 a charge to the coroner's jury read: "Gentlemen

[25]Virginia Magazine of History and Biography, v. 4, p. 185.
[26]Ibid., v. 5, p. 40.
[27]Surry County Records, v. 1, p. 194.

of the Jury yo are to make diligent enquiry How Robt Whittell came to his death. . . . And to Cause all psons bystanding to touch the sd Corps & to retourne yr verdict accordingly. . . ." The jury found that he died by accident.[28]

For his services the Virginia coroner was well paid. An act of 1677 provided that "Forasmuch as some doubts have arisen concerning coroners ffees in this colony, and it being necessary to declare by a law what the same shall be, Bee it therefore enacted by the Governour, Councell and Burgesses of the present Grand Assembly, and the authority thereof, and it is hereby enacted, that a ffee for a coroner's inquest be thirteene shillings and ffowre pence according to the allowance in England in such cases, or one hundred thirty three pounds of tobacco and casque at the choice of the coroner to be paid out of the estate of the person deceased, if such there be, and for want of such estate by the county where the party causeing the inquest shall dye, and where there is noe coroner in the county, that the justice of the peace doeing the office shall have the ffee."[29]

In 1691 an autopsy was held on the body of Governor Slaughter of New York. Toner[30] and others consider this the earliest American necropsy. Packard[31] records six autopsies in New England between 1674 and 1678. Ball[32]

---

[28]Surry County Records, v. 1, p. 234.
[29]Hening: Statutes at Large, v. 2, p. 419.
[30]Toner: Contributions to the Annals of Medical Progress and Medical Education in the United States, 1874.
[31]Packard: History of Medicine in the U. S., p. 62.
[32]Ball: The Sack-'Em-Up Men, p. 198.

quotes Hartwell's find of a manuscript account of two chirurgeons viewing the head of Benjamin Price, supposed to have been killed by the Indians. Long before any of these, autopsies had been performed in Virginia. On April 28, 1624, George Menefie wrote from Jamestown to John Harrison in England, describing how Harrison's brother, George, died "fourteen days after a duel with Richard Stephens, in which he received a small cut in the knee only; the jury at the inquest, after a post-mortem examination, affirmed that he died of natural disease."[33] In the Northampton (Accomac) County Records, 1636, we have the deposition of John Wignall that "he heard Capt. Howe tell John Holloway yt he would give nothing ffor opening ye corps of Mr. Christopher Thomas, & yt he ye sd Howe said yt John Hollaway had need to give him 500 wt. of tobaccoe to gayne experience."[34]

IV

Parish Medicine

The parish was an important political as well as ecclesiastical unit in "Episcopal Virginia." Before 1662 the vestry, usually consisting of twelve men, was elected by the people, but after that date by act of the Assembly it became a closed, self-perpetuating corporation with distinctly oligarchical tendencies. The counties and parishes overlapped

---

[33]Calendar British State Papers, v. 1574-1660, p. 61.
[34]Northampton County Records, v. 5, p. 124.

politically as well as geographically. In 1680 there were twenty counties, fifty parishes and thirty-seven ministers. The powers of the vestry were as extensive as those of the justices who presided over the counties. They made up the parish budget, apportioned and collected taxes, elected the minister, church wardens and clerk, supervised the counting of tobacco, processioned "the bounds of every man's land," and were the sole overseers of the poor.

It was in this last capacity that the vestry touched the medical profession. The charity patients of each parish were the special charge of the vestries, who appear to have been consistently careful of this social responsibility. The vestry books, especially that of Christ Church, Middlesex County, contain interesting medical items and give the names of many early doctors. Various physicians were paid, and paid well, to treat the indigent sick, and often the patient was sent to the doctor's house "for to live" while under treatment, the expense of "diett, washing, lodging and apparell" being paid for out of the parish levy.

From the Parish Register of Christ Church we learn that William Poole, chirurgeon, had a wife named Sarah, that his son was christened in 1668, and that he himself died February 29, 1687. The vestry book shows him attending the poor of the parish from 1678 to 1685. At a vestry meeting November 5, 1678, "It is ordered that Mr. William Poole, chirurgn, to be paid for his Attendance and pains taken about ye cure of Robt Main, 2000" (pounds of tobacco).[35] He was not so successful with another patient, who was blind, but he received a thousand pounds of tobacco for his effort.

Dr. Robert Deputy, whose two marriages are recorded in the Parish Register, was offered by the vestry 2,000 pounds of tobacco in 1699 to cure Ellianor Slanter, a parish charge.[36] Dr. Tankerly, 1696, was paid by the vestry for "administring Physick to a poore man."[37] Dr. Thomas Stapleton in 1684 and 1693, and Dr. William Oastler in 1697, were rewarded for similar services.[38] Mention is made of Dr. Rose, 1667, and of Dr. Whittaker, 1671.

Dr. Robert Boodle, whose marriage to Elizabeth Best in 1685 and whose children's births in 1688-1691 are recorded, was frequently employed by the vestry to visit the poor of Middlesex County. An order of 1690 "that mr. Robert Boodle be paid for keeping a bastard Child, omitted last Yeare" shows the vestry and the physician cooperating in the solution of an only too common social problem. An entry dated November 12, 1688, illustrates the pains taken to reach a fair decision in a doubtful case. "It is ordered by this present Vestry That ye present Church-Warden of ye Lower Prcinq namely mr. Matthew Kemp Doe Take into his Custody and Care a poore Decripped & lame Wo-

[35]Vestry Book, Christ Church Parish, p. 28.
[36]Ibid., p. 88.
[37]Ibid., p. 81.
[38]Ibid., pp. 45, 75, 83.

man Named Bridgett Press Causeing her to be Conveyed to Dor. Boodle and to have his Judgement about her lameness and that ye Said mr. Kemp and mr. Robert Dudley are by us directed to advise and agree wth ye Said Dor. Boodle or any other able Doctor or cirurgion about her Cure."[39]

---

[39]Vestry Book, Christ Church Parish, p. 60.

Chapter X

VOCATIONS AND AVOCATIONS

I

Ship Surgeons

EVERY ship that crossed the Atlantic in the early days faced the certainty of sickness and death among passengers and crew. Many captains were glad to shift this responsibility to the shoulders of their ship surgeons. These men must have represented a great variety of training and skill. Most of them, doubtless, were poorly educated, with nothing to recommend them for their calling but a smattering of drugs, a little practice in opening abscesses and a liking for the sea. A few probably had gone through the schools. They were usually chirurgeons. Their pay was fair and they ranked fourth among ships' officers in the distribution of the spoils of sea warfare, being superceded only by the Captain, Lieutenant, Master and Mates.[1] Captain Smith defines their duties and qualifications: "The Chirurgeon is to be exempted from all duty, but to attend the sicke, and cure the wounded: and good care would be had he have a certificate from Barber Chirurgions Hall of his sufficiency, and also that his chest be well furnished both for Physicke and Chirurgery,

---

[1]Smith: A Sea Grammar, p. 296.

and so neare as may be proper for the clime you goe for, which neglect hath beene the losse of many a man's life."[2]

Ship surgeons were both a blessing and a curse to the medical profession. In New Amsterdam it soon became necessary to regulate them by law, and the Council handed over to Dr. Montague the authority to issue permits under which they might practise in the colony: "Ship barbers shall not be allowed to dress any wounds nor minister any potions on shore, without the previous knowledge and special consent of the petitioners, or at least of Dr. Montague." Dr. Montague was also charged with the responsibility of passing upon Barber Surgeons who applied as ship surgeons on out-going vessels.[3] This regulation of the colonial practice of ship surgeons had apparently no counterpart in Virginia, though the same necessity for some sort of control must have existed. The Swiss traveler, Michel, was taken sick as he was about to leave Virginia for Europe. Knowing that the ship in which he had come over was at Yorktown, he wrote, ". . . I rather preferred to go to my old Captain . . . Besides, the doctor, a Saxon, was my friend and the ship was better supplied with provisions than any other ship in the fleet."[4]

Some ship surgeons gave up the sea and settled in the colony. John Edwards, of the Eastern Shore, was prob-

_____

[2]Smith: A Sea Grammar, p. 258.
[3]Walsh: Medicine in N. Y., p. 33. (From a Dutch Record, Feb. 2, 1652.)
[4]Virginia Magazine of History and Biography, v. 24, "Journey of Michel to Virginia."

ably one of these, for at his death in 1667 he still held a
share in the Ship *Susan,* and his name appears in county
records of Northampton and Lancaster off and on for a
decade. Some of them practised here only when their ships
were in port. They were apparently much sought after by
the sick, who found doctors both scarce and expensive in
their neighborhoods and who probably looked upon the
surgeon on a ship just out of European waters as the exponent of the latest medical practice. Some settled in the colony
and years later took to the sea again. The names of a few
of these men, with a hint of romance forever fastened to
them by their adventurous calling and by the picturesque
names of their ships, have survived: Henry Hitch of the
James, Samuel Mole, Raphael Shemans of the *Great Hopewell,* and Richard Walters, "Doctr of Moore's ship" (the
Assurance of Bristol), who is mentioned by William Fitzhugh in 1692.[5] Thomas Fawn made his will as he was
about to sail for Virginia on Christmas Day in 1651, and
left a watch and cornelian ring to Robert Williams, surgeon
of the Virginia trading ship, *Peter.*[6] One Jacobs, ship surgeon, went to court in 1679 to recover a stolen hat. James
Love, who was apparently the surgeon on board the *Alexander,* bequeathed to the commander of that ship his
"wages, Surgery Chest, & other chest. . . ."[7]

There was likewise Thomas Levett, "Chirurgeon of the
Ship *Endeavour,*" who was called into court to testify for

---

[5]Virginia Magazine of History and Biography, v. 3, p. 372.
[6]Neill: Virginia Carolorum, p. 219n.
[7]Rappahannock County Records, v. 7, p. 90.

his Captain in a dispute;[8] Maurice Jones, "of the Shipp Golden Lyon;" and Thomas Burn, surgeon on the *Young Prince,* who was in Virginia waters during Bacon's Rebellion and kept a journal of the events of that stirring time.[9] Robert Eedes, "Chirurgion of ye Hopewell," figured in a controversy which resulted in the master of his ship paying to one Henry Catelyne, "Marchant," "Six pounds of lawfull mony of England for the passage of a maide whom the said Chirurgion hath married since her arrivall in this Country."[10] Henry Bysant, boatswain of the *Marmaduke,* and William Kidwell, a sailor, swore in Court that "Richard Hewes, their Chirurgion, did say . . . that when one boy of Mr. Cappes was goeing ashoare at ye Cowes, hee would warrant his comeing aboard againe & ye boy came aboard againe."[11] Dr. James Montgomery, of the man-of-war *St. Albans,* died in Richmond, England, about 1697 and left his property in Virginia to his two brothers.[12] With these scattered bits of information we must piece together the pattern of the colorful life of the ship surgeon three centuries ago.

II
Explorers

Virginia had some notable explorers among her early physicians. In the Eighteenth Century there were Thomas

---

[8]York County Records, v. 6, p. 272.
[9]Calendar British State Papers, v. 1675-76, p. 454.
[10]Minutes of Council and General Court, p. 160.
[11]Ibid., p. 134.
[12]York County Records, v. 1657-62, p. 118.

Walker, the pioneer to Kentucky, and Christopher Robinson, who was one of Spottswood's Knights of the Golden
Horse Shoe.

Virginia's first and most intrepid explorer was Captain
John Smith. Two physicians took part in his excursions into
the interior of Virginia. Dr. Walter Russell was in the first
expedition and rendered professional services to the party,
besides saving their lives with his timely warning of
Opechancanough's treachery. Anthony Bagnall was associated in "the second Voyage in discovering the Bay."

In 1634 there was a certain Mr. Scott, a physician, who
accompanied Captain Thomas Young's expedition of exploration to America. Captain Young had secured a pass
for himself, his nephew, Robert Evelin, and Mr. Scott, to
be employed by the king in America upon "special and
weighty affairs concerning private service."[13] They planned
to search the unexplored parts of Virginia and adjacent
regions. In April 1634 Young wrote to Secretary Winde-
bank that the party had "already given satisfaction to his
majestie, in swearing their Allegiance." In July of the
same year, they landed at Point Comfort. Subsequently
they visited Jamestown before proceeding to explore the
Delaware River.[14]

Another explorer was Dr. Woodward, a famous Indian
Trader, who is said to have travelled up by the Indian paths
from Carolina to Virginia in 1671.[15]

---

[13]Calendar British State Papers, v. 1574-1660, p. 177.
[14]Neill: Virginia Carolorum, p. 105.
[15]William and Mary Quarterly, v. 2, second series, p. 235.

E Catalogo huc tranfmiffo *Anno* 1680. quem compofuit
eruditiffimus Vir & confummatiffimus Botanicus
D. *Johannes Banifter* Plantarum à feipfo in Virginia
obfervatarum.

A.

ALfine Spergula latifolia reptans.
Becabunga folio.
Althæa lutea Pimpinellæ majoris folio, floribus
parvis, feminibus roftratis. Folia hujus plantæ
pediculis infident.
Althæa magna Acoris folio, cortice Cannabino,
floribus parvis femina rotatim in fummitate
caulium, fingula fingulis cuticulis roftratis co-
operta ferens.
Althæa magna quinquecapfularis, cortice Cannabino, foliis integris fubtus albicantibus, floribus magnis ex fundo faturatè rubro albis.
Alth. magna quinquecapfularis, cortice Cinna-
bino, foliis Malvarum modo divifis, fubtus viridibus.
Ambrofia inodora foliis non divifis.
giganrea inodora foliis afperis trifidis. ,
Anchufa lutea minor, quam Indi Paccoon vocant
feipfos ea pingentes.
Anemone latifolia fylveftris alba.
Apocynum erectum non ramofum folio fubrotun-
do, umbellis florum rubris.
Apoc. erect. non ramof. latiore folio, umbellis
florum albicantibus.
Apoc. erect. minus, umbellâ florum candida.
Apoc. erect. non ram. Afclepiadis folio, umbellis
florum rubentibus.
Apoc. minus non lactefcens, caule & foliis hirfu-
tis, floribus faturatè luteis.
Apoc. erect. non ram. Roris marini foliis umbel-
lis florum candidis.
Apoc. petræum ramofum Salicis folio.
Apoc. fcandens, capfulis brevibus fpinis afperis.
Apoc. fcand. capfulis alatis.
Apoc. fcand. capfulis planis.
Hæc omnia filiquas ferunt tumentes.
Apoc. erect. ramofum, caule rubente, foliis ob-
longis parvis, filiquis [ex flofculis albis] tenu-
iffimis, binatim ad extremitates conjunctis.
Arifarum triphyllum, pene viridi.
Arif. triph. minus, pene atro-rubente.
Arif. Dracontii foliis pene longo acuminato.
Arum aquaticum, foliis in acumen definentibus,
fructu viridi.
Arum flutans, pene nudo.

C.

Carduus Jaceoides purp. foliis fubtus incanis, capite vifcofo.
Caryophyllata flore femper albo.
Caftanea pumila racemofo fructu parvo, in fingula capfulis echinatis unico, The Chinqua-
pin. Autor defcriptionis Carolinæ ex hac
nuce Chocolatam fieri refert non multò inferi-
orem ei quæ ex Cacao fit.
Centaurium minus caule quadrato alato, flore
carneo amplo, umbilico luteo.
Centaurium luteum Alcyroides.
Clematis purpurea repens petalis florum coriaceis.
Clem. erecta, humilis non ramofa, folus fubrotundis, flore unico ochroleuco.
Cochlearia flore majori In locis udis à falfis
procul remotis. .

Conyza cœrulea acris Americana.
Cucumis fructu minimo viridi, ad maturitatem
perducto nigricante. Fructus Bryoniæ albæ
baccâ non multo major eft, cujus primo afpectu
fpeciem effe putaveram.

D.

Dens caninus flore luteo.
Digitalis flore pallido tranfparenti, folus & caule
molli hirfutie imbuta.
Digit. rubra minor, labiis florum patulis, foliis
parvis anguftis.
Digit. lutea elatior Jaceæ nigræ foliis.
lutea altera, foliis tenuiis diffectis thecis
florum foliaceis.
parva comis coccineis.

E.

Eryngium campeftre Yuccæ foliis, fpinis tenellis
hinc inde marginibus appofitis.
Euonymus capfulis eleganter bullatis.

F.

Filix mas foliis integris auriculatis.
mas rachi feu nervo medio alato.
fœmina foliis per margines pulverulentis,
feminibus fimbriatis.
Fumaria filiquofa lutea.
Siliquofa altera grumofa radice, floribus
gemellis ad labia conjunctis.
Fungus (ex ftercore equino) capillaceus capitulo
rorido, nigro punctulo in fummitate notato.
Ex recenti fimo noctu exoritur cauliculis erectis, vix digitum longis, capillorum inftar tenu-
bus nec minùs dentis feu confertis. Singuli
Cuiiculi parvulo globulo aqueo coronantur,
qui in fumma fui parte macula parva nigra Limacis oculo fimili infignitur.

G.

Gentianæ affinis foliis glabris ferratis, floribus Ra-
næ referentibus.
Gladiolus cæruleus hexapetalos, caule etiam gla
diato.
Gratiola foliis latioribus ferratis.

H.

Hedera trifolia Canadenfis foliis finuatis.
Helleborine flore rotundo luteo, purpureis venis
ftriato. The Mockafine flower.
Helxine latè fcandens feminibus majoribus.
Helxine frutefcens Bryoniæ nigræ foliis, capfulis
triquetris amplis Pergamenis.
Hieracium fruticofum latifolium foliis punctulis
& venis fanguineis notatis.
Hyacinthus Occidentalis flore pallide cœruleo.
Hypericum parvum caule quadrato feu Afcyron
minimum.
Hyper. pumilum femper virens caule compreffo
ligneo ; ad bina latera alato, flore luteo terra-
petalo, feu Crux S. Andreæ.
Hyper. frutefcens luteum Phillyrheæ foliis.

Jicea

Banister's Catalogue of Virginia Plants, in Ray's *Historia
Plantarum*.

I.

Jacea non ramofa tuberofa radice, foliis plurimis rigidis peranguftis, flores ferens multos parvos rubentes acaules in fpica ad caulem feffiles.

Jac. non ram. tub. rad. foliis latioribus flores ferens pauciores, majores, fquamis hiantibus armatos & pediculis curtis infidentes.

Jacobæa lanata foliis brevibus fubrotundis, lanata altera foliis longis anguftis.

Jafminum arboreum foliis amplis, oblon.gis, fupernè virentibus, fubtus leni canitie pubefcentibus, flores albos in quatuor lacinias longas anguftas ad umbilicum ufque partitos racematim ferens.

Iris aculeata baccifera arborea minùs ferax.

Iris cœrulea latifolia & anguftifolia.

Chamæ-Iris verna odoratiffima, latifolia cœrulea repens.

L.

Pfeudo-Lathyrus luteus glaber,filiquis tumentibus, duplicem feminum feriem continentibus.

Pfeudo-Lath. lut.hirfutus filiq. tument.continentibus duplicem feriem feminum.

Laurus Tinus floribus albidis eleganter bullatis. Flos nondum apertus pyxidi S. M. Magdalenæ (ut nonnunquam pictam vidi) fimilis eft.

Lilio-narciffus humilis albus.

Lilium S.Martagon floribus reflexis ex luteo rubentibus, purpureis maculis eleganter notatis.

Lilium S. Martagon pufillum florib. minutiffimis herbaceis. Caulem habet vix dodrantalem,verticillo foliorum unico cinctum, cujus fummitas quatuor floribus reflexis Solani lignofi floribus magnitudine haud æqualibus, pediculis parvis infidentibus coronantur.

Lilium Squillæ foliis, denticellis parvis ad margines ferratis. Caule eft alto, nudo, ad cujus fummitatem prodeunt flores in fpica feffiles, petalis pæne ad imum (ut loqui amant feciales) quafi erafis; ftaminibus fex (fi non malè memini) purpuro-cœruleis, mole fua aliquantulum depreffis. Flos quamvis afpectu non admodum pulcher fit pergratum habet odorem. Radicem habet imbricatam inftar Lilii, folia craffa admodum & fucculenta, non tamen Sempervivi fpecies eft.

Lonchitis maxima foliis planis *i. e.* non dentatis, nec pulverulentis maculis notatis, uno in cefpite foliorum unicum protrudens caulem foliis anguftioribus, pulverem feu femina in membranulis quafi in capfulis ferentibus compofitum.

Lonchitis major Polypodii facie. Hæc atque etiam vulgaris fimili modo florida eft.

Lychnis plumaria alba, foliis ad geniculum quatuor cruciatim pofitis, thecis florum tumentibus.

Lyfimachia lutea minor, foliis & floribus purpureo punctatis.

Lyfimachia filiquofa lutea minor.

M.

Meliffa elatior foliis magnis dentatis glabris, ad geniculum binis: flores odoratos luteos patulos ftamina bina quafi cornua protrudentibus in fummitate caulium racematim ferens.

Mercurialis tricoccos hermaphrodicæa, f. ad foliorum juncturas ex foliolis criftatis Julifera fimul ac fructum ferens.

Mufcus erectus denfè complicatus Cupreffi foliis major & minor. In rupe quadam prope Sabinas foliis Cupreffi.

Myrrhis minor procumbens, feu potiùs Cerefolium.

N.

Nux veficaria Virginiana *Park.*

O.

Orchis palmata elegans lutea cum longis calcaribus luteis, palmata lutea minor nullis calcaribus. Hermaphrodicica, flore minore, calcare longiore.

Origanum floribus amplis luteis, purpureo maculatis, cujus caulis fub quovis verticillo decem vel duodecimo foliis eft circumcinctus.

Orig. cujus ramorum fummitates floribus dilutè rubris in verticillos congeftis coronantur.

Orig. foliis ad fummitatem caulium canis, floribus multis pallidè cœruleis in cymis ramorum denfè ftipatis.

Ornithogalum luteum parvum foliis gramineis hirfutis.

Orobanche radice dentata caule & flore albo. Flos ejus quem unicum in uno caule Goodyeri Orobanches fimilis eft fed major. Conceptaculi feminalis venter feu pars protuberans non rotunda eft fed canaliculata.

P.

Pepo fructu parvo compreffo.

Phalangium ramofum floribus albis, ad fundum viridibus.

Phalangium album non ramofum floribus albis ad caulem fpicatim feffilibus.

Phyllitis parva faxatilis per fummitates folii prolifera.

Pifum fpontaneum purpureum.

Plantago aquatica latiore folio.

Polygala feu Flos ambarvalis floribus luteis in caput oblongum congeftis.

Polyg. rubra fpicà parvà compacta.

Polygala fpicata rubra major foliis & caulibus cœrulefcentibus.

Pol. quadrifolia S. cruciata floribus ex viridi rubentibus, in globum compactis.

Pol. quadrif. minor fpica parva rubente.

Polygonatum ramofum capfulà prifmaticà, ramofum perfoliatum flore ochroleuco capfula trigonà.

Polypodium parvum foliis minutim ferratis.

Polypodium minus alterum Scolopendriæ facie.

Potamogiton Virginianum.

Q.

Quercus variæ fpecies, 1.Pumila. 2. Alba. 3. Rubra. 4. Hifpanica. 5. Caftaneæ folio. 6. Lini aut Salicis foliis. 7. Fruticofa. Harum primam in Hiftoriæ, quintam in Appendice memini mus.

R.

Ranunculus Thalictri folio, radice grumofa; Anemone fylv.

Rapuntium minimum glabrum. In uliginofis minùs glabrum flore pallidiore.

Rhamnus Prunifolius fructu nigro, officulo compreffo. **The black Haw.**

Rhus ramis ex ftipite pullulantibus glabris. Hujus truncus carpi craffitiem nunquam fuperat, pollicis raro excedit. Baccæ fapore funt fubfallo cum pungenti illo acore qui in Tamarindis fentitur mixto.

Rubia parva foliolis ad geniculum unumquodque binis, flore cœruleo fiftulofo.

· **Aaaaaaaa** 2   Rub.

Banister's Catalogue of Virginia Plants, in Ray's
Historia Plantarum.

Rub. parvâ latifolia foliis ad genic. binis, flore rubente.

S.

Sanicula feu Auricula urfi Cyclamini flore.
Saxifraga petræa Altinefolia.
Sedum faxatile parvum, caule gracili aphyllo, floribus rubentibus.
Solanum verticillatum latifolium molle, floribus obfoletè rubris, baccis luteis.
Sol. verticill. anguftiore folio, flore ochroleuco.
Sol. triphyllum flo. tripetalo, atro-purpureo, in foliorum finu abfque pediculo feffili.
Staphis agria fol. dilutè viridibus.
Stramonium fundo floris cœruleo, pomis longioribus fpinis armatis.

T.

Trichomanes major foliis longis auriculatis.

U.

Valeriana Græca feu Valeriana cœrulea minor.
Veronica pratenfis Serpyllifolia.
Viola tricolor nudo caule, foliis tenuius diffectis.
Viola alabaftrites pentaphyllea, Cochleariæ fapore, Nafturtii fpecies.
Urtica urens major feminibus rotundis, compreffis loculamentis viridibus inclufis & in caulis fummitate racematim difpofitis.

Inter femina ad me ê Virginia tranfmiffa, *Anno* 1687. ab eodem *D. Banifter*, nonnulla invenio quorum nomina *in hoc* Catalogo non habentur, v. g.

Erigeron (frutex marit.) Halimi folio : Senecio arborefcens Atriplicis folio.
Eryngium Plinii Portulacæ foliis à *D. Spragge* acceptum.
Euonymus (ni malè memini) Pyracanthæ folis.
Lyfimachia lutea corniculata maritima.
Cynogloffum cœruleum Bugloffi foliis.
Senæ fpuriæ tres fpecies quarum una filiquis eft hirfutis à *D. Spragge* acceptæ. Duæ à me fatæ germinârunt & plantas produxerunt, quæ duæ fpecies Paiominobæ à Pifone defcriptæ effe videbantur.
Piftacia nigra Coryli folio *D. Spragge.*
Ulmus fructu Lupulino.
Ricinus parvus Urticæ folio.
Convolvulus bicapfularis feminibus pappo alatis.
Phalangium fpicatum flofculo Arbuteo bullato aureo.
Lithofpermum floribus roftratis.
Ricinus frutefcens Fici foliis.
Gramen marinum echinatum. Hujus femina etiam a *D. Spragge* accepi, quæ hac æftate in horto fata germinârunt, fed nondum ad frugem pervenerunt.

C O M-

Banister's Catalogue of Virginia Plants, in Ray's *Historia Plantarum.*

The discoverer of Fauquier County was John Lederer. Thomas Glover, an "ingenious Chirurgeon," wrote of Lederer in 1676: "About five years since there was a German Chirurgeon who obtained a Commission from Sr. Will. Bartlet to travel to the southwest of Virginia to make discovery of those parts."[16] In 1672 we find "Doctor Liderer" mentioned in the records of Surry County. He was probably the same chirurgeon-discoverer.

John Lederer appears to have come from Germany to this country and to have landed a stranger at Jamestown, proposing explorations to study the Indian inhabitants, their lives, manners and characteristics. He was well read in American history, spoke the Italian, French and English languages and was a master of the classics. Hearing of Governor Berkeley's desire to explore the mountains, he offered his services and was sent on three separate overland expeditions to the Manahoac country from the neighborhoods of Yorktown, Richmond and Fredericksburg respectively. On a second journey he claimed to have gone as far south as Florida, but was deserted by his companions. On his return he was abused and persecuted. Mobs were instigated against him, and he fled to Maryland, where Governor Sir William Talbott befriended him and secured the publication of his experiences as *The Discoveries of John Lederer in Three Several Marches from Virginia, etc., March, 1669-Sept. 1670.* This is the first description of the

---

[16]Philosophical Transactions of the Royal Society, June 20, 1676, Oxford reprint, 1904.

geography of the Alleghany mountains. On the last journey he was accompanied by Colonel John Catlett, "with nine English horse and five Indians on foot."

Lederer's account is entertaining but has little in it to suggest that it was written by a physician. Even his experience with a mountain spider shows him helplessly relying upon the services of an "Indian Doctor." "Here I was stung in my sleep by a Mountain-spider; and had not an Indian suckt out the poyson, I had died: for receiving the hurt at the tip of one of my fingers, the venome shot up immediately into my shoulder, and so inflamed my side, that it is not possible to express my torment. The means used by my Physician, was first a small dose of Snake-root-powder, which I took in a little water: and then making a kinde of Plaister of the same, applied it neer to the part affected: when he had done so, he swallowed some by way of Antidote himself, and suckt my fingers end so violently, that I felt the venome retire back from my side into my shoulder, and from thence down my arm: having thus sucked half a score times, and spit as often, I was eased of all my pain, and perfectly recovered. I thought I had been bit by a Rattle-snake, for I saw not what hurt me: but the Indian found by the wound, and the effects of it, that it was given by a Spider, one of which he shewed me the next day: it is not unlike our great blue Spider, onely it is somewhat longer, I suppose the nature of his poyson to be much like that of the Tarantula."[17]

---

[17]Ratterman: John Lederer's Discoveries, 1669-1670.

Ratterman, who in 1879 published Lederer's *Discoveries* in English, says that little is known of him. There was a Lederer who wrote a geographical description of the Alps in 1691, and a family of Lederers taught at the University of Wittenberg in the Sixteenth and Seventeenth Centuries. As with other discoverers there have been people who questioned whether John Lederer ever saw the mountains and who claimed that the narrative he left "looks like fiction, the working up, no doubt, of Indian traders' talk."[18]

III

Parson Physicians

The exigencies of an age that interpreted sickness and death as part of the retributive justice of an overruling spirit produced the Shaman, who was both priest and doctor. The alliance, often unholy, continued, with a break here and there, well through the Middle Ages. To the Church and the monasteries medicine owed much—hospitals, nursing, the preservation of the Greek texts, and some great medical schools, such as Salerno. The new learning and the appreciation of the force of natural phenomena made the breach, though the stamp of the theological bias lingered in the respect which men like Culpeper and Paracelsus paid to magic, charms and incantations. The Vicar of Stratford-on-Avon wrote in the Fifteenth Century that, "In King Richard II's time physicians and divines were not

---

[18]William and Mary Quarterly, second series, v. 1, p. 234.

distinct professions, for one Tydenian, Bishop of Landolph and Worcester, was physician to Richard II."[19]   Studies of Jewish physicians in Italy and elsewhere have shown the frequency with which men have been both physician and rabbi.[20]

The parson-physician was common in all the colonies. Preachers came to the new world with the missionary spirit and prepared themselves to save bodies as well as souls.   In New England there were notable examples, among them John Fisk, John Rogers and Thomas Thacher, the first minister to the Old South Church in Boston.

Two "zieckentroosters," who were really visitors of the sick, came to New Amsterdam from Holland and held divine service every Sunday until the arrival of the minister. They appear to have given both spiritual and physical consolation, though they apparently had had little experience in medicine.   In 1628 the Reverend Jonas Michaleius arrived and combined the practice of medicine with ministerial functions.   New York had no regular physician until 1637.

In Virginia the same custom prevailed.   It continued well into the Eighteenth Century, when Mrs. Washington called on the Reverend Greene, M. D., for medical advice.   The earliest Virginia minister who was also a physician was the Reverend Robert Pawlett.   He arrived in 1619 and settled at Martin's Hundred.

Nathaniel Eaton was an early minister who added a

---

[19]Haggard: Devils, Drugs and Doctors, p. 188.
[20]Personal communication from Dr. Henry Friedenwald.

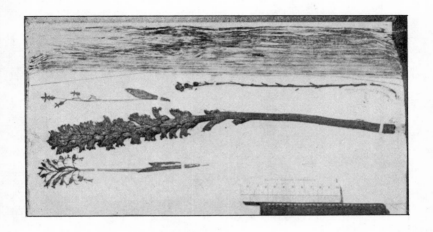

Cancer Root. An actual specimen from Banister's *Hortus Siccus,* with the
description in his handwriting.

degree in medicine to his other titles. He was a restless, maladjusted individual, spending most of his life wandering from England to America and back again, frequently in trouble, and finally dying in a debtors' prison. He was born in 1609, son of the Vicar of Great Budworth, a pensioner at Trinity College, Cambridge, and Scholar from Westminster. In 1632 he obtained a license to go to Leyden. From Holland he went to New England to become the first principal of Harvard College. He was the brother of the Governor of New Haven. Debarred from teaching on account of cruelty, he absconded to England and came to Virginia in 1639 as assistant to the Reverend John Rosier, of Northampton County. Here he married Anne Graves. In 1646 he again fled to England. A desire for learning overtaking him once more, he repaired to Padua, where he took the degrees of Ph. D. and M. D. He became Vicar of Bishop's Castle, Shropshire, and later Rector of Bedeford in Devonshire, returning no more to America.[21]

John Banister, though a minister of the Church of England, was also an enthusiastic naturalist and entomologist. After traveling in the West Indies he came to Virginia, probably as a missionary, and was living in Charles City County as early as 1678.[21a] In 1690 he held grants of land

---

[21]Goodwin: Colonial Church in Virginia, appendix.

[21a]John Banister "gave up his place as professor of botany and librarian at the University of Oxford, and settling in Virginia, at great pains and with rare judgment, collected and described a number of scarcest plants." (Count Castiglioni, quoted in A. J. Morrison: Travels in Virginia in Revolutionary Times, p. 65.)

in Bristol Parish. He followed his scientific studies vigorously in Virginia and made several notable contributions to the botany of the colony. He was a correspondent of a number of distinguished scholars of the day, among them Ray, Compton, who was Bishop of London, and Martin Lister, who called him "my friend Mr. Banister, a very learned and sagacious naturalist." His *Catalogue of Virginia Plants* was published in Ray's *Historia Plantarum,* and his collection of plants is now in the British Museum. Other writings of Banister were *Curiosities in Virginia, On Several Sorts of Snails, Insects of Virginia, Descriptions of the Snake Root* and *Observations on the Natural Products of Virginia.*[22] He died in 1692. His death is usually attributed to a fall from rocks on Roanoke River while he was on a botanical trip, but Henrico County records show that Jacob Colson was arrested "for the death per misadventure of Mr. John Banister" and was later acquitted. It is probable that the minister was accidentally shot by Colson.[23]

Another clergyman with a strong taste for science was John Clayton, minister at Jamestown from 1684 to 1686.[24] He was a friend of Robert Boyle, and several of his letters, written to Boyle from Virginia, have been preserved. In

---

[22]Encyclopedia of Virginia Biography, v. 1, p. 179; William and Mary Quarterly, second series, v. 4, p. 244n; Philosophical Transactions Royal Society, 1690-93, v. 17, p. 667.

[23]Virginia Magazine of History and Biography, v. 11, p. 164.

[24]John Clayton, famous botanist of the next century, was not his son, but the son of John Clayton, attorney general of the colony.

one he speaks disparagingly of Virginia physicians and asks advice in case he should contract "gripes" (lead poisoning), then prevalent in the colony. In a letter to the Royal Society, May 12, 1688, he gives an account of several observations in Virginia: "In September the Weather usually breaks suddenly, and there falls generally very considerable Rains. When the weather breaks many fall Sick, this being the Time of an endemical Sickness, for Seasonings, Cachexes, Fluxes, Scorbutical Dropsies, Gripes, or the like which I have attributed to this Reason. That by the extraordinary Heat, the Ferment of the Blood being raised too high, and the Tone of the Stomach relaxed, when the Weather breaks the Blood palls, and like overfermented Liquors is depauperated, or turns eager and sharp, and there's a crude Digestion, whence the name Distempers may be supposed to ensue. And for Confirmation, I have observed the carminative Seeds, such as warm, and whose Oil sheaths the acid Humors that ever result from crude Digestions. But Decoctions that retain the Tone of the Stomach, as I suppose, by making the little Glands in the Tunicles of Stomach, squeeze out their Juice, (for what is bitter may be as well offensive to the Stomach, as to the Palate) and then Chalibiates that raise the decayed Ferment, are no bad Practice. . . ."[25]

Clayton was evidently a keen observer, but like many others was not able to distinguish between *post hoc* and

---

[25]Force: Tracts, v. 3, Letter of John Clayton, p. 6.

propter hoc: "Tis wonderful what influence the Air has over Men's bodies, whereof I had my self sad Assurances; for tho' I was in a very close warm Room, where was a Fire constantly kept, yet there was not the least Alteration or Change, whereof I was not Sensible when I was sick of the Gripes, of which Distemper I may give a farther Account in its proper Place. When a very ingenious Gentlewoman was visited with the same Distemper, I had the Opportunity of making very considerable Observations. I stood at the Window, and could view the Clouds arise: for there small black fleeting Clouds will arise, and be swiftly carry'd cross the whole Element; and as these Clouds arose, and came nigher her Torments were encreased, which were grievous as a labouring Womans; there was not the least Cloud but lamentably affected her, and that at a considerable Distance; but by her Shrieks it seemed more or less, according to the Bigness and nearness of the Clouds."[26]

The reverend scientist had a strong belief in the effect of air upon the human constitution and attributed sickness to the inland reaches of salt water: "So far as the salt Waters reach the Country is deemed less healthy. In the Freshes they more rarely are troubled with the Seasonings, and those endemical Distempers about September and October. This being very remarkable, I refer the Reason to the more piercing Genius of those most judicious Members of the

---

[26]Force: Tracts, v. 3, Letter of John Clayton, p. 7.

Society: And it might perhaps be worthy the Disquisition of the most Learned to give an Account of the various Alterations and fatal Effects that the Air has on Humane bodies, especially when impregnated with a marine Salt, more peculiarly when such an Air becomes stagnant: This might perhaps make several beneficial Discoveries, not only in Relation to those Distempers in America, but perhaps take in your Kentish Agues, and many others remarkable enough in our own Nation. I lately was making some Observations of this Nature, on a Lady of a delicate Constitution who living in a clear Air, and removing towards the Sea-Coast, was lamentably afflicted therewith, which both my self and others attributed to this Cause, she having formerly upon her going to the same, been seized in the same Manner."[27]

Clayton made some significant observations on the urine, advocated the oil of tobacco in the treatment of indolent sores, and had firm convictions about the efficacy of snake stones for snake bite and about volatile salts, as a vomit, for dog bite. He approved of the Indian method of treating snake bite and described how a savage, bitten between the fingers by a snake, "stretched his Arm out as high as he could, calling for a String, wherewith he bound his Arm as hard as possibly he could, and clapped a hot burning Coal thereon, and singed it stoutly, whereby he was cured, but looked pale a long while after. And I believe, this truly one

[27]Force: Tracts, v. 3, Letter of John Clayton, p. 12.

of the best ways in the World of curing the Bite either of Viper or mad Dog."[28]

He gives many examples of how he has successfully handled hydrophobia. One of his cases had a relapse: "It was a relapse of its former Distemper, that is, of the Bite of the mad-Dog. I told them, if any thing in the World would save his Life, I judged it might be the former Vomit of volatile Salts; they could not tell what to do, nevertheless such is the Malignancy of the World, that as soon as it was given, they ran away and left me, saying, he was now certainly a dead Man, to have a Vomit given in that Condition. Nevertheless it pleased God that he shortly after cried, *this Fellow in the Black has done me good,* and after the first Vomit, came so to himself, as to know us all. I vomited him every other day with this Vomit for three times, and made him in the interim to take volatile Salt of Amber, and the aforesaid Powders, and to wash his Hands and Sores in a strong salt Brine: to drink Posset-Drink with Sage and Rue, and by this Course, and the Blessing of God, his Life was saved and he perfectly cured, for it was now four Years since, and he had had no Relapse. I have cured several others by the same Method."[29]

The Reverend Francis Makemie was described by the Governor of New York in 1704 as "a preacher, a doctor of physick, a merchant, an attorney and what is worst of all a disturber of government." He was born near Rathmelton,

---

[28]Force: Tracts, v. 3, Letter from John Clayton, p. 39.
[29]Ibid., v. 3, p. 43.

Ireland, in 1658, studied for the ministry at Glasgow University, and came to America in 1681, with misionary zeal. The Barbadoes, Maryland and Virginia were all scenes of his activities. He settled in Accomac in 1690 and married Naomi, the daughter of William Anderson. He formed the first Presbytery in America, organizing it in 1706. His preaching took him far afield. At Newton, Long Island, he was arrested and fined for preaching without a license. He died in 1708 in Accomac County and is regarded as the father of Presbyterianism in America.[30]

IV

Physicians as Lawyers

That the legal profession in the colony of Virginia was at first held in somewhat low repute is shown by a series of statutes regulating lawyers. The first of these was passed in 1642/43. All "mercenary attorneys" were expelled from their offices because they "more intended their own profit and their inordinate lucre than the good and benefit of their clients." Soon after this it was enacted that attorneys "shall not take any recompense" for appearing in court.

Both on account of these restrictions and because of the simple nature of most of the early law business there was little encouragement to trained lawyers, and we find the more prominent citizens—merchants, planters and physicians—acting as attorneys and pleading causes in the courts.

---

[30]Wise: Eastern Shore, p. 281.

In 1666 the debts of Captain Richard Longman, filed in York County court, include these two items:

"To Mr. Robt Ellyson as attorney agt Jones at
   James City & the County Court...........10-00-00"
"To Dr. Robert Ellyson for physicke in my sick-
   ness 1663............................12-00-00"[31]

This is the same Robert Ellyson who appears at other times as Captain, Sheriff and Burgess.

Still more versatile was Daniel Parke, physician, planter, merchant, colonel, justice of the peace, burgess, councillor, Secretary of State, and, as the following entry shows, lawyer as well: "Geo. Lee, Cittizen and Grocer of London" in 1662 appoints Daniel Parke his "true and lawfull Attorney, Factor & Agent" in Virginia.[32]

Another doctor-lawyer was "Tho: Culmer of Surry County Chyrurgion," to whom Walter Turner wrote in 1661:

"Loving friend Doctor Culmer: I desire you that you would do me the favour at Court as to crave a refference untill ye next Court in the suite of Peckes between him & I. Soe I rest etc. ...."[33]

In 1674 we find this letter from Roland Plan to Dr. George Lee, a Surry County physician:

"Doctor Lee: Having sevrall actions to come before yor

---

[31]York County Record, v. 4, pp. 114, 117.
[32]Ibid., v. 3, p. 429.
[33]Surry County Records, v. 1, p. 185.

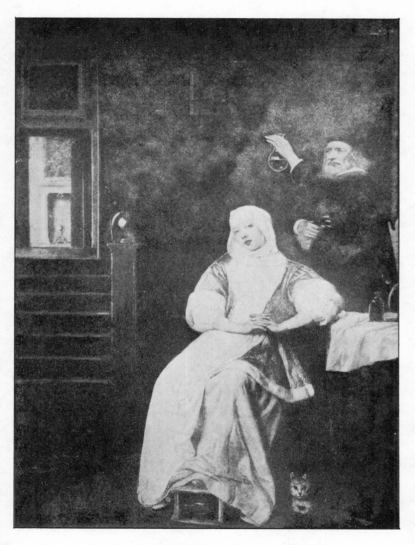

Dutch painting, illustrating uroscopy.

Cort lett me beg the favour to implead all the parties at my sute, yor haveing at present what papers is requisite. . . ."[34]

Between 1664 and 1667 the Rappahannock County records show that "Geo. Davis phisitian" was three times appointed attorney to represent different people in court.[35] Many similar instances might be given, for they occur frequently in all the county records. The Reverend John Clayton summed up the situation fairly accurately when he wrote from Virginia in 1684, "They have few scholars so that every one studys to be halfe physitian halfe lawyer & wth a naturall accutenesse would amuse thee for want of bookes they read men the more. . . ."[36]

V

Foreign Doctors

Although Virginia was settled by English stock, trade and adventure must have brought to her shores foreigners from friendly countries, some of whom remained to make a home. When home talent failed, the English sought in other countries specialists in the several industries they wished to introduce into the colony. Poles and Dutch were sent over to operate the glass works, and when these did not succeed Captain Norton imported skilled workmen from Italy. France contributed the vine-dressers. It is not surprising,

[34]Surry County Records, v. 2, p. 59.
[35]Rappahannock County Records, v. 2, p. 96.
[36]William and Mary Quarterly, Second Series, v. 1, p. 114.

therefore, to encounter a number of alien nationalities among the early physicians in the colony. The scarcity of doctors made necessary frequent appeals to England, and explains the welcome given those foreigners who were escaping unbearable conditions in their own lands.

Among the German physicians who emigrated to Virginia was John Lederer. His reputation was chiefly made as the explorer of Fauquier County, but he probably also practised medicine in Surry County.

George Hacke, born in 1623, settled in Northampton County in 1653 and received a grant of 100 acres. He is described as "docr George Hacke, Practiconr in Physicke, a high German (both by parents and birth), borne in ye Citty of Collyne [Cologne] under the Palatinate." His wife was Anne Herman, a native of Amsterdam. In 1653 Dr. Hacke had the Court declare him a German, possibly in order not to be thought a Dutchman, since there was considerable hostility against the Dutch because of England's war with Holland. The Journals of the House of Burgesses record Dr. Hacke's attempts to have himself and his family naturalized: "Denization issued in the forme above specified to George Hacke, Chirurgeon, being a German borne, now resident in the County of North'ton . . . ," and later, "Whereas George Hacke had formerly a Commission of denizacon granted him in the year Sixteen hundred fifty-eight, And hath petitioned in behalfe of himselfe, his Brother & Children yt the same might be renewed to him & Conferred on Them. The Grand Assembly hath thought fitt to grant Confirmation thereof on his & their takeing ye oathes of Allegiance & Sup'macie."[37]

In 1661 a duel was fought on the Eastern Shore between Gosling Van Nerson and a servant of Christopher Calvert. The servant received the worst of the affray, and the court ordered Calvert to pay Dr. George Hacke, who had apparently been summoned to treat the servant.

Dr. Hacke paid for the passage of a number of immigrants to Virginia in 1652 and 1653.[38] When he died, he left a large library, written chiefly in German, and a thousand acres of land in Ncrthampton County.[39] His son, Peter, was a justice of Northumberland in 1699 and a member of the House of Burgesses in 1706, later becoming colonel of Northumberland militia.[40] The other son, George Nicholas, was appointed Sheriff of Accomac County in 1700.[41]

John Williams was an out-and-out Dutchman and a chirurgeon, serving out his indenture. Perhaps because of the hostilities with the Low Countries life was so unpleasant for him in Virginia that he attempted to escape to New Amsterdam. For this attempt the court ordered him "after his full time expired with his master to serve the Colony seven years."[42]

[37]Journals House of Burgesses, v. 1619-58, pp. 112, 131.
[38]Greer: Early Virginia Immigrants, pp. 109, 363, 364.
[39]Bruce: Institutional History of Virginia, v. 1, p. 432.
[40]Virginia Magazine of History and Biography, v. 5, pp. 37, 257.
[41]Executive Journals, Council of Colonial Virginia, v. 2, p. 46.
[42]York County Records, v. 4, p. 188.

Among the French physicians who settled in Virginia was one who signed himself "John Peteet, Sirurgione." He appears in the records between 1657 and 1670. We find him in 1666, like other foreign-born physicians, seeking naturalization: "Whereas John Petit a frenchman by birth but an ancient inhabitant of this country wherof his marreage children long abode many service & approved fidelity have justly made him reputed a member hath peticoned . . ." that he be made "Denizen to this Country," it is granted by the Governor, Council and Burgesses that he be made a free Denizen of "this his Ma^{ts}es Countrey of Virg^{a}."[43] He was a large importer of servants and had extensive holdings in land. Like many of his contemporaries he was frequently in court, suing and being sued. He appears to have charged high fees, for a deposition of Thomas Jackson declares that Charles Allen "cured him of that as Mr. Peteet would not have done it for 1000 lbs. of tobaccoe."[44] His will, dated December 1669 and filed April 26, 1670, begins "I John Petit of Yorke pish in the County of Yorke, chirurgion," and leaves five shillings to each of his daughters. The rest of his estate, "housing, lands, mares, cattle, househould stuffe, Servants," he leaves to his "loving wife Rebecca Petit," who is made sole executrix.[45]

Dr. John Jacob Coignan Danze, whose name suggests his French origin, is found between 1668 and 1698 paying

---

[43]York County Records, v. 4, p. 399.
[44]Ibid., v. 3, p. 232.
[45]Ibid., v. 4, p. 399.

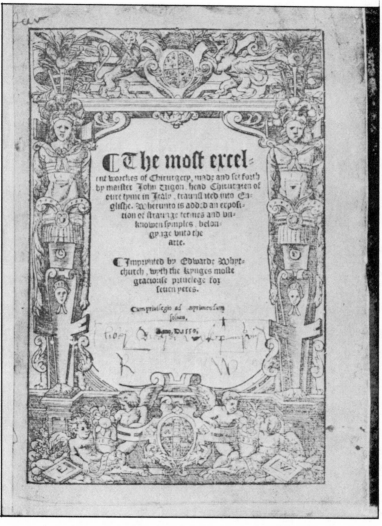

Title page of Vigo's *Surgery,* a book often found in
Seventeenth Century Virginia libraries.

professional visits and administering "Physsicall Meanes" to the citizens of York County.[46]

Peter Plovier, whose wife in 1666 signed her name "ffranchois a Pluvier," was a chirurgeon and evidently a Frenchman.[47] He practised in York County between 1659 and 1678. His will in 1677 disposed of a feather bed, a heifer and the rest of his estate "to my loving wife Elizabeth Plouvier." Characteristic of the times, the loving wife married before his will was probated, and the new husband, John Griggs, probated the will and collected the debts due his predecessor. Several years later we find Elizabeth, now the wife of Thomas Nutting, disposing of 100 acres formerly belonging to "Peter Plover."[48]

Dr. Giles Modé was also a Frenchman, whose name was corrupted to Moody and who is the founder of the Virginia family of that name. He lived in York County and brought in a number of immigrants. The Journal of the House of Burgesses records in 1654: "Upon the petition of Dr. Gyles Moody & John Mitchell & other strangers—Inhabitants of this Country It is ordered that the aforesaid persons be made denisons to purchase & hold any lands & Priviledges here (offices & publick employment excepted). . . . Nevertheless all Children of such strangers within Limitted or any other shall upon suite by them made Obtaine Denizacon."[49]

---

[46]York County Records, v. 8, pp. 236, 338, 389, 411; v. 9, pp. 207, 241, 409; v. 11, p. 336; v. 12, p. 48.
[47]Ibid., v. 4, p. 135.
[48]Ibid., v. 6. p. 50; v. 8, p. 19.
[49]Journals House of Burgesses, v. 1619-1658, p. 95.

Dr. Modé was a Justice of York County in 1655 and died in December 1657, leaving a rather large estate, including a library "all written in the Dutch language." His widow, Jane, soon married another physician, Francis Haddon, who became administrator of Dr. Modé's estate and guardian of his three sons, Josias, Humphrey and Philip.[50]

Still another Frenchman was Dr. John Montone, who practised medicine in Northumberland County. Though he had lived in Virginia for twenty years and was one of her substantial citizens, he found it necessary in 1663 to declare emphatically his abhorrence for the Romish Church. He certified that he was a "frenchman by birth hath lived in this countrey 20 yeares, a great part of which time in this county, and hath demeaned himselfe like an honest & industrious man, and it hath pleased god for to bless his labour & industry that hee hath purchased a small parcell of Land, living conformable & obedient to his Maties Lawes & Edicts, & declares himself to adhere to and imbrace the true Protestant Religion & utterly denying & abhorring the Rites & superstitious Ceremonies of the Romish Church wherefore he most humbly implores that by the Supreme authority of this Countrey he may be made capable of the abilitys of his Maties subjects & enjoy his enfranchizement & Denization."[51]

There is a curious reference to a Mousnier de la Montagne whose name heads a list of "such Wallons and French as offer themselfs to goe into Virginia" and who is described

[50]York County Records, v. 1, p. 62; v. 2, pp. 25, 56; v. 3, p. 444.
[51]Northumberland County Order Book, March 8, 1663, p. 193.

as "medical man; marrying man." The date was probably
1621, and the document states: "We promise my Lord
Ambassador of the Most Serene King of Great Britain to
go and inhabit in Virginia . . . as soon as conveniently may
be."[52] These French and "Wallons" probably never came
to Virginia. "Mousnier de la Montagne" may have been
the same person who signed himself "Jean de la Montagne"
at the University of Leyden in 1619.[53] This Jean, a Huguenot, born at Saintonge, was a refugee to Holland, studied
medicine at Leyden, and in 1639, at the age of forty-four,
emigrated to New Amsterdam where he became a distinguished physician. He married prominently, was a friend
of Governor Stuyvesant, was appointed by the Council to
supervise the medical practice of ship surgeons, and took a
prominent part in opposing the massacre of the Indians in
1642 in New York. Dr. Pott, under similar circumstances
in Virginia, instead of opposing, apparently aided and
abetted the killing of the Indians.

Another interesting foreigner was Dr. Siccary, a Portuguese Jew, said by Thomas Jefferson to have introduced the
tomato into this country. The authority for this statement
cannot be found. The love apple, as the tomato was formerly called, belonged to the night shade family (solana-
ceae), was reputed to be poisonous, but was used medicinally. Prejudice against it was due to the confusion of the
woody night shade with the deadly European night shade,

[52]Calendar British State Papers, Addenda, 1574-1660, p. 498.
[53]Walsh: History of Medicine in N. Y., v. 1, p. 19.

which contained belladonna. The accepted belief is that
the tomato was first introduced into the United States from
South America just prior to 1830.

There are surprisingly few Scotch and Irish names among
the early Virginia doctors. The two Napiers, Patrick and
Valentine, were Scotch physicians living in York County.
Patrick was apparently prosperous and upon his death in
1669 left 1,500 acres in New Kent County to his wife,
Elizabeth, the daughter of Dr. Robert Booth, of York
County.

In 1661 we find Patrick Napier in court, involved in one
of the petty disputes over fees which marked the medical
practice of the time. During the trial Napier asks the defendant, Mrs. Graves, the following questions: "(1)
Whether you did not send for Patrick Napier in February
last to Administer meanes to yor Selfe and one Mathew. . . .
(2) Whether you did not after you were recovered to yor
health agree to pay mee for ye meanes I administered. . . .
(3) Whether you afterwards did not agree with mee for
Five pounds sterl to season your new hands." Mrs. Graves
replied "Noe" to the first two questions, and to the third
she said, "I told him that hee should not middle with mee
till that he had agreed with my Father for ye year. . . ."
Mrs. Graves's servant then testified that "being sent over
to Mr. Patrick Napier by his Mrs. Rachel Graves . . . to
bring with him some meanes for hir legge & to take away
his feaver the said Napier Swoare God Damne him hee had

MEDICAMENTS
FOR THE
POOR;
OR,
PHYSICK
For the Common People.

'In Two BOOKS,

I. Containing excellent Remedies for moſt Common Diſeaſes, incident to Mans Body; made of ſuch
things as are common to be had in almoſt every Countrey
in the World; and are made with little Art, and ſmall
Charge.

First written in Latin by that famous and learned Doctor, John Pre-
votius, *Philoſopher and publick Profeſſor of Phyſick in Padua,*
Tranſlated into Engliſh, with additions.

SECONDLY,

HEALTH
FOR THE
RICH and POOR,
BY
DIET, without PHYSICK.

By Nich. Culpeper, *Student in Phyſick and Aſtrology.*

LONDON,
Printed by JOHN STREATER, for *George Sawbridge*
dwelling on Clerkenwell-green, 1670.

Title page of Culpeper's *Medicaments for the Poor,* often found in
Seventeenth Century Virginia libraries.

done as much as hee could unto hir & that hee could doe noe more. . . ."[54]

VI

Veterinarians

Animal experimentation has played a large part in the development of medicine, and the study of animals and their diseases has naturally interested many physicians. Most of the ancient anatomy and physiology was based entirely on observation of animals. Zoroaster required the physician to treat animals as well as human beings. The dog in particular was to receive the same drugs as a rich man. The English have long recognized the importance of comparative anatomy and the study of diseases common to man and beast, and their medical curricula prescribe compulsory courses in veterinary medicine.

Throughout the Seventeenth Century English books gave evidence of improvement in veterinary medicine and surgery, especially in the treatment of the horse. In 1683 Andrew Snape, farrier to Charles II, brought out his famous *Anatomy of an Horse*. In the same century de Solleysel demonstrated that glanders could be transmitted from one horse to another.

On both sides of the water stress was laid on live stock, and in colonial Virginia the services of veterinarians were sought and valued. William Carter was an expert veterinarian, or cow doctor, who lived in James City in 1625. In

[54]York County Records, v. 3, p. 376.

a lawsuit in that year, being sworn and examined, he "sayeth That he drest a Cow for Mr. Allnutt in May last was twelvmonth for wch demandinge 10 s.   Mr. Allnutt did not pay him, And the last springe there was A Cow ... with a fistula uppon the Eye ... and about Easter last he offered Mr. Allnutt ... to cure ye cow wth ye fistula for 20 s. in money soe as he might be satisfied for the former cure, wch Mr. Allnutt refused saying he had rather give another man forty shillings then him 20 s. and so put the Cow to goodman Tree's man to Cure, who not beinge to cure her Mr. Allnutt offered this deponent to give him content yf he would Cure her ..." Carter accordingly "used his best skill, yett at length she dyed."[55]

In 1670 Thomas Willkinson wrote: "Coll Jordan: pray you be pleased to assist me in my busines of Mr. Geo Lee's for I cannot possably be over for my Cattle are all very pore & Crasey...."[56]

Dr. John Holloway is found in 1642 marking the ear of a calf for Thomas Smyth.[57]   In York County Thomas Spilman was awarded 400 pounds of tobacco from John Smith, who had sent Spilman his horse "to use the best of his skill for the cure of the horse."   The animal died, but the owner was "at the opening of the horses wound" and brought no charges of lack of skill, so the court decided that he must stand the loss and pay for the treatment.[58]

---

[55]Minutes of Council and General Court, p. 85.
[56]Surry County Records, v. 1, p. 380.
[57]Northampton County Records, v. 1640-45, p. 159.
[58]York County Records, v. 6, p. 44.

Butler suggests in his *Hudibras*,

"That there was a time
When cattle feel indisposition
And need the opinion of a physician."

No doubt this often happened in Virginia.

VII

Physicians in Business

Along with his varied public activities the physician had his own business interests to look after. We find him frequently importing servants and patenting land. The records show that Dr. Henry Lee brought in seven servants. Dr. Robert Synock paid for the passage of eight persons, Dr. Richard Hall for six, Dr. John Severne five, Dr. John Holloway ten, and Dr. William Bankes three. Everyone in Virginia was vitally interested in land and in the cultivation of tobacco. The parson grew the crop on the glebe, and the physician divided his time between agriculture and his patients. The importation of servants was intimately bound up with the acquisition of land, since fifty acres was the reward for paying the passage money of a new settler. John Peteet brought in twenty-three persons and acquired 1,150 acres.[59] Daniel Parke, by paying the passage money of thirty-one servants, added 1,550 acres to his estates.[60]

[59] York County Records, v. 3, p. 114; v. 4, p. 250.
[60] Ibid., v. 5, p. 168.

John Overtstreet was granted a certificate for 250 acres for transporting five persons to Virginia.[61]

Now and then business took the Virginia doctor to Europe. Richard Townshend made repeated voyages between 1635 and 1647. Thomas Blake, of James City County, crossed in 1693.[62] The York County records preserve the statement of John Toton, May 1632, that "the subscriber intends for England this shipping."[63] Peter Hopegood in May, 1678, "Being in health and perfect memory . . . and Intended for England and considering the Dangers of the seas . . ." prudently makes his last will and testament before departing.[64]

---

[61]York County Records, v. 4, p. 138.
[62]Ibid., v. 9, p. 381.
[63]Ibid., v. 6, p. 407.
[64]Rappahannock County Records, v. 7, p. 71.

CHAPTER XI

MEDICAL FEES

I

Money Values

HE landed estates, slaves and great families usually associated with colonial Virginia belonged to the Eighteenth rather than to the Seventeenth Century. Before 1700 the small land owner of the English yeoman class predominated, and slavery made little headway until the end of the century. The first rent rolls of the Public Record Office in London show that thousands of little proprietors, with holdings of from fifty to five hundred acres, constituted the largest part of the colony.[1] Travel was difficult, labor high, and clothes precious; houses were small and usually made of wood; and during most of the century the price of tobacco was depressed. There was plenty of food and freedom, but little real wealth, as the will and deed books of the counties sufficiently prove. Notwithstanding the general lack of opulence there is much evidence that the doctors and chirurgeons of the century demanded and received substantial fees—fees that astonish us when translated into present day values.

---

[1]Wertenbaker: Planters of Colonial Virginia, pp. 52, 53.

As a matter of fact there has seldom been a time when physicians have not been well paid. The code of Hammurabi, 2250 B. C., fixed medical and surgical charges in Babylon. Ten shekels of silver, worth about $600 today, was the fee for treating a severe wound, and five shekels for curing "diseased bowels."

In Greece the honorarium of the physician varied from the equivalent of twenty cents to one hundred dollars a visit. Their municipal physicians received salaries equal to about $2,000 a year. Cleombrotus is said to have been paid the unique fee of $100,000. At Rome the average physician made thirty cents a visit. When the difference in the purchasing power of money is considered, this is the equivalent of a modern fee. There were Roman physicians whose yearly income exceeded $25,000. Even in the Middle Ages fees were high. One-half of a tarrene of gold "for each day's service" was the medical tariff imposed by the law of the Emperor Frederick II (1194-1250).[2] The tarrene was equal to five dollars today. At about the same time in England the distinguished surgeon, John Arderne, was getting the equivalent of $500 for his fistula operation. In the Fourteenth and Fifteenth Centuries in Venice a physician's fee for a visit ranged from twelve to twenty soldi.

In 1605 the Duke of Rutland paid Mr. Peck thirty shillings for letting blood, and in 1679 the accounts of the same

---

[2]Huillard-Brehallis: Diplomatic History of Frederick II.

family show "to my Lord 12 dayes 12£"—a pound a visit, paid to Dr. Harwood.[3] An Irish physician of the Seventeenth Century, Thomas Arthur, has left an interesting fee book. In 1619 for a cure of gonorrhoea he collected in advance 2£, equivalent to fifty dollars now; for assisting a patient "in escaping putrid sore throat," eight shillings; for a case of orthopnea, six shillings. Early in his practice his earnings for about ten months netted 74£ 1s 8d, or $2,000 today. Later, in 1632, his annual income averaged between $6,000 and $7,000.[4]

The expression of money values in shekels, tarrenes, soldi and shillings is confusing, and direct comparisons of values are impossible.[5] Our interest centers on the purchasing power of money. We find that in Babylon the fee for setting a fracture would hire a day's laborer for six months. A city visit in the Middle Ages netted the equivalent of the wages of two laborers for a day. In Venice in the Fourteenth and Fifteenth Centuries a laborer would have to work two days to pay for a doctor's visit. In England a day's work was worth four pence—just the price of a pair of shoes; a fat goose could be had for 2½d, a sheep for 2s 2d, and an ox for sixteen shillings.[4]

The same principle of using the cost of the common commodity as a standard must be adhered to in considering the

---

[3]Lancet, London, 1915, p. 1213.
[4]Walsh: N. Y. Medical Journal, 1912, xcvi, pp. 370-373.
[5]Rogers: History of Agriculture and Prices in England, v. 5. p. 675, says that 2s. in the 17th Century had the value of $2 in 1895. Today those values should probably be doubled.

fees of the Seventeenth Century Virginia physician. The Virginia laborer was six or seven times as well paid as his contemporary in England, because labor was very scarce in the colony. George Sandys said that in 1623 the Virginia laborer got a pound of tobacco a day, with food, when tobacco was worth three shillings a pound. Mechanics demanded extraordinary pay—three to four pounds of tobacco a day, with food. In 1649 the annual wages of a laborer ran from three to ten pounds.[6] Bullock calculated that if these wages were prudently invested in certain trading operations which he describes, one could amass sixty pounds in four years. In 1680 wages were on a parity with England's—a housekeeper receiving passage, food and three pounds annually.[7] In 1695 a seaman received by the month 2£ 4s, the chief mate 4£, the ship's physician 3£ 10s, and the ship's carpenter the same. The average horse sold for 600 pounds of tobacco, but a bay gelding in York County brought 2,000 pounds and a mare 3,360 pounds in the latter half of the century. A negro slave sold for from 2,100 to 3,600 pounds of tobacco. A broadcloth coat cost 240 pounds of tobacco and a bushel of corn 150 pounds in 1620. In 1625 butter by the firkin was twenty pounds, wine by the gallon brought three pounds, and a pound of sugar was worth a pound of tobacco. Land varied from thirteen to sixty-six pounds of tobacco an acre. Coffins sold for from 60 to 250 pounds of tobacco, the grave-digger

[6] Bruce: Economic History of Virginia, v. 2, pp. 48-51.
[7] Ibid., v. 2, pp. 48-51.

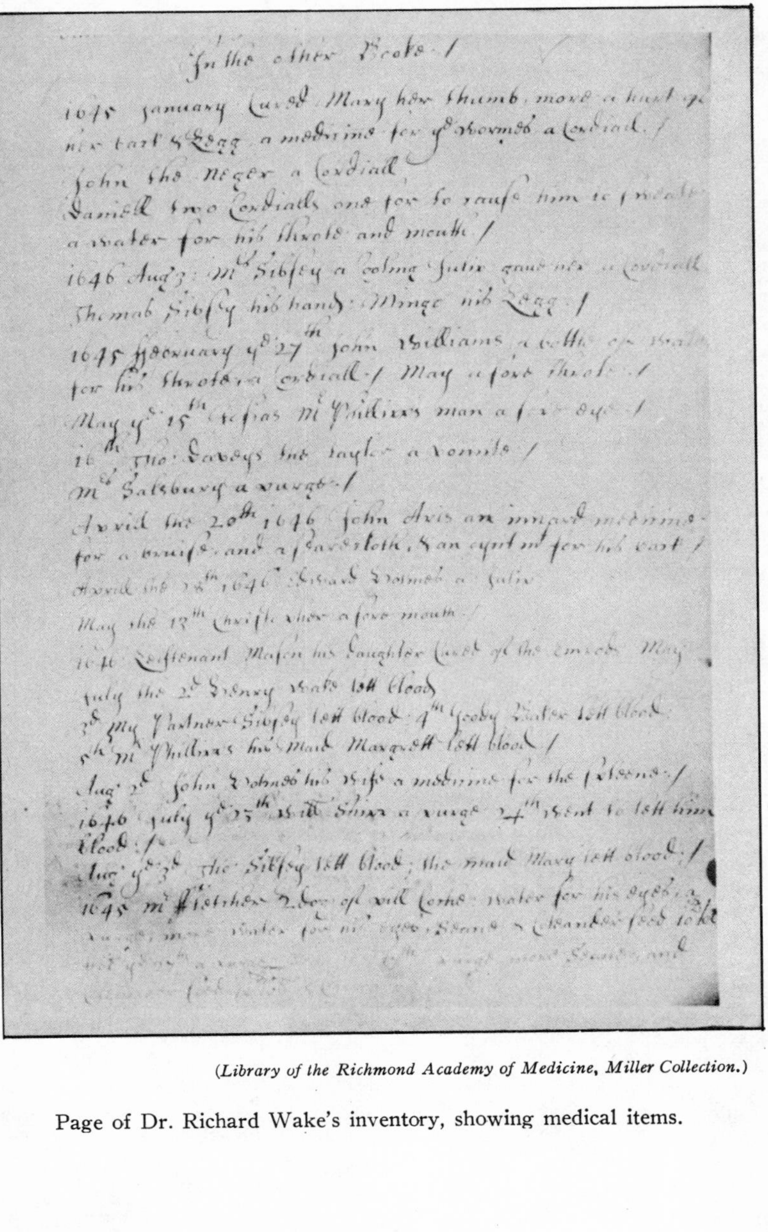
In the other Booke /
1645 January Cured Mary her thumb, more a hurt of
her eare & Legg a medicine for ye wormes a Cordiall /
John the Negro a Cordiall
Daniell two Cordialls one for to cause him to sweate
a water for his throate and mouth /
1646 Aug 3: Mrs Sibsey a cooling Julip and her a Cordiall
Thomas Sibsey his hand: Mingo his Legg /
1645 ffebruary ye 27th John Williams a bottle of water
for his throate a Cordiall / May a sore throate /
May ye 15th Tobias Mr Phillips man a sore eye /
16th Tho: Davys the taylor a vomite /
Mrs Salsbury a purge /
April the 20th 1646 John Avis an inward medicine
for a bruise and a seare cloth, & an oyntment for his eare /
April the 28th 1646 Edward Holmes a Julip
May the 13th Christopher a sore mouth /
1646 Leiftenant Mason his daughter Cured of the [illegible] May
July the 2d Henry Wake lett blood
3d My Partner Sibsey lett blood 4th Goody Baker lett blood
5th Mr Phillips his Maid Margrett lett blood /
Aug 2d John Holmes his wife a medicine for the [illegible] /
1646 July ye 23th Will Shaw a purge 24th went to lett him
blood: [illegible]
Aug ye 3d Tho: Sibsey lett blood; the maid Mary lett blood /
1645 Mr ffletcher 2 doz of [illegible] water for his eyes a
purge, more water for his eyes [illegible]
[illegible]
[illegible]

(Library of the Richmond Academy of Medicine, Miller Collection.)

Page of Dr. Richard Wake's inventory, showing medical items.

charged 30 to 60 pounds of tobacco for his services, and
the funeral sermon cost from 200 to 400. Lawyers charged
100 pounds of tobacco for writing a will, and 50 pounds
was a marriage fee.[8] In 1679 the Governor received
120,000 pounds of tobacco annually, the Chaplain 16,000,
and the Chirurgeon 11,000.[9]

Virginia had practically no specie in the Seventeenth
Century, and a primitive system of barter prevailed. The
scarcity of coin was deplored and legislated against, but
there was little improvement until after 1700. Toward the
end of the century some specie was to be found, chiefly
Spanish, Arabian, French, Portuguese, Dutch and New
England coins. As late as 1701 Michel wrote, "There is
little money in the country, the little that is found there
consists mostly of Spanish coins, namely dollars. Tobacco
is the money with which payments are made."[10] Debts
were paid with anything that had value, even with hens and
beaver skins. There are many instances of corn being used.
In 1636 Dr. John Holloway was awarded a barrel of corn
in a law suit, and in 1642 Dr. Stringer paid a debt in corn.
The real medium of exchange was tobacco, a bulky commodity with a fluctuating value. It encouraged indebted-
ness and made for much litigation to settle obligations.

During the first three decades of the century Virginia

---

[8]The above prices of commodities are taken from inventories in the
county records of York, Surry, Henrico and Rappahannock.
[9]Virginia Magazine of History and Biography, v. 24, p. 364.
[10]Ibid., v. 24, "Journey of Michel to Va."

produced less than 500,000 pounds of tobacco annually, and the price remained around three shillings a pound. After this production greatly increased, so that by the end of the century thirty-eight ships were yearly exporting more than 15,000,000 pounds. The consequence was that from 1630 to 1700 the price of tobacco took a great drop and rarely exceeded three pence. The average for the greater part of the century was two pence.

PRICE OF VIRGINIA TOBACCO IN THE 17TH CENTURY[11]

YEAR	PRICE	YEAR	PRICE
1617	5s 3d	1644	1½d
1622	2s	1655	2d
		1657	3d
1624	3s	1664	1d
1627	3s 6d	1667	½d
1630	1d	1685	2d
1640	6d	1695	1½d

II

Medical and Surgical Bills

Under the London Company the Physician-General was paid by the Company. Dr. Bohun was allotted "500 acres of land and 20 tenants to be placed thereon, at the Company's charge," and Dr. Pott came over under the same arrangement. Earlier physicians, Wotton and Russell, undoubtedly received their pay through the Company, for

[11]Summarized from Bruce: Economic History of Virginia.

during the first years everything was in common, and medical attention was furnished free. Yet even before 1624 doctors had probably begun to render personal bills for their services.

The following items give a fairly good idea of the charges made by the Seventeenth Century physician. Francis Haddon was paid 400 pounds of tobacco "for 6 visitts, my coming by night watching & attendance. . ." in 1660, when a laborer could produce from 800 to 1,000 pounds of tobacco in a year.[12] George Wale, for three visits and five days' attendance, received 300 pounds of tobacco.[13] Another physician in York County rendered a bill for 1,000 pounds "to twenty daies attendance going ounce a weeke . . . being fourteen miles," and 600 pounds for "12 daies going to his own house at the Middle plantation"—50 pounds a visit.[14] Dr. John Toton, of James City, "desired that it might be recorded . . . That hee would not visitt at their request any Person lying sick in York County unless the person he did visitt would give him ten shillings ster: for each visitt."[15]

Surgical procedures were not elaborate in those days, but the pay was good. Dr. Irby received three pounds sterling in 1684 for setting a thigh,[16] while Dr. Robert Ellyson for "reducing" a shoulder asked 600 pounds of tobacco.[17] The

---

[12]York County Records, v. 3, p. 203.
[13]Ibid., v. 3, p. 67.
[14]Ibid., v. 4, p. 444.
[15]Ibid., v. 6, p. 354.
[16]Henrico County Records, v. 2, p. 170.
[17]York County Records, v. 3, p. 329.

cure of a burnt hand was considered worth 80 pounds of tobacco; putting up a rupture, 50; a phlebotomy, a frequent item, usually cost 20 pounds, and cupping was done for the same price. Glisters (enemata) were regularly 30 pounds.

Drugs, which were scarce and expensive, were usually dispensed by the physician and charged for separately. Favorite prescriptions were billed as follows: a laxative bolus, 20-50 pounds of tobacco; an astringent, 20-35; opiate pills, 30-100; a cordial, 30-50; a "very rich one," 80; an electuary, 30-40; juleps, 50-120; defensives, 20; ointments, 10-40.

The county records show many medical items in the settlement of estates. From 1637 to 1700 the medical bills in York County records alone number 145. The average of all these bills is 752 pounds of tobacco, a little less than one laborer could produce in a year, more than the value of a horse or an ox. The charges range from a few pounds of tobacco up to 3,300 pounds, the cost of a good slave. They represented probably a month of service for "physical means and attendance." Doctors' visits were not made for trivial causes in those days, and the physician was probably not called until the disease was well declared and serious.

A few of these bills rendered at the end of an illness should be cited. In Rappahannock County in 1686 Dr. William Brasey asked 400 pounds of tobacco from the estate of Nathaniel Grubb for "physical means administered to him in his sickness." William Thornbury received

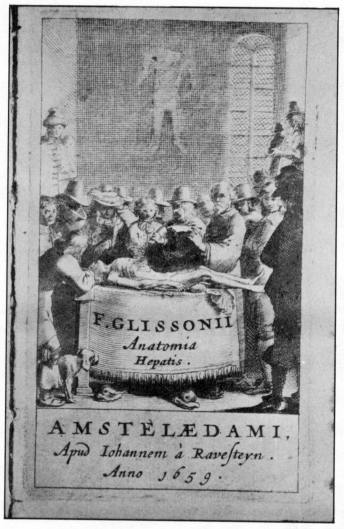

F. GLISSONII
Anatomia
Hepatis.

AMSTELÆDAMI,
Apud Iohannem à Ravesteyn.
Anno 1659.

Title page of Glisson's *Anatomy,* often found in Seventeenth
Century Virginia libraries.

the same amount from Cornelius Williams "uppon acct physical means administered." In 1684 William Bendry owed Dr. Synock 500 pounds of tobacco, "due upon Chirurgery Accompt." In 1682 the estate of William Gray was indebted to Drs. Synock, Russell and Poole for a total of 1,500 pounds of tobacco. In 1684 Dr. Richard Pemberton rendered a bill against Thomas George for 900 pounds of tobacco "for Physical means administered." The same year Dr. Robert Clark presented a bill to Robert Handley for 850 pounds of tobacco, "due for physical means Administered to the sd Hendley in the time of his sickness." In Henrico County in 1678 Dr. Spears and Dr. Cagan each rendered accounts for 1,000 pounds of tobacco against the estate of Mrs. Elizabeth Epes, while Dr. Irby's bill against the same estate amounted to only 300 pounds of tobacco. In Elizabeth City County in 1684 Dr. William Ellis entered suit against the estate of William Harris for "7 lb. 10s. sterl. money acct of Medicines, visits, advice & attendance in time of his sickness." In 1677 the bill of Dr. Francis Taylor against Mr. Chambers for 552 pounds of tobacco was presented in Surry County court and ordered paid. In 1643 Dr. John Stringer received from the estate of N. Palmer of Northampton County 400 pounds of tobacco. In 1633 we find Dr. John Holloway collecting a bill for administering "phisack to Lady Dale's and Mr. Throgmorton's servants, 750 lb. tob." The following is the bill of Dr. Giles Modé, rendered June 30, 1657, against George Light of York County :[18]

"An electuary with vomiting	030
A glister & Administering	050
A phlebotomy to Jno Simans	020
A cordiall	030
A glister & Ad.	050
A dose of physick	050
A julip	025

July 4

A phlebothany to yr Mayd	020
A laxative sirrups	020
Stomack powdrs	40
. . . .	30

——— (pounds of
415" tobacco)

Dr. John Clulo presented the following :[19]

His bill to John Gosling, March 22, 1658 :

"For 2 glisters	040
" a glister	030
" a potion Cord.	036
For an astringent potion	035
For my visitts paines & attendance	. . .
For a glistere	030
For an astringent potion	035
For a cord. Astringent bole	036
For a bole as before	036

---

[18]York County Record, v. 2, p. 69.
[19]Ibid., v. 3, p. 66.

For a purging potion   050
For a cordyall Iuleb   120
For a potion as before   036
                           ——— (pounds of
                      1284   tobacco)
              Allowed   1084
         (Signed)   John Cluloe"

Patrick Napier's account against the estate of Jarves reads:

"To the cure of a Cancer in his mouth   150
to 1 Bottle Cordiall Apoz: 100
to phlebt.   020
to 1 Bottle Julepp   030
to 1 Cordiall pt   060
to 1 phlebt.   020
to 2 dose Cordiale Spet   120
to 2 Dose Cordiall Spts   100
to ungt for side   010
to 1 Cordiall Mago   100
to pect meens   010
to ungt for side   010
to my paynes & attendance   300
                           ——— (pounds
                      1060"   tobacco)[20]

III
Bargaining

Bargaining between doctor and patient was common. The patient wanted assurance of a cure. The expenditure

---

[20]York County Records, v. 4, p. 144.

of a doctor's time and skill was considered worth something, but the cure was worth more, and it was often so stipulated. In 1683 Dr. William Poole, of Middlesex County, was promised 2,000 pounds of tobacco for curing a case of blindness. If he failed he was to have only "reasonable satisfaction for his trouble."[21] John Toton was rash enough to contract to cure Robert Prichard "in a fortknight time" for 40 shillings, the equivalent at that time of 240 pounds of tobacco.[22] Dr. Peter Plovier made a unique bargain with Thomas Kirby and family, of "Warrwicke County." He promised to administer "such Phisick, Medicines and Chirurgery as hee or any of his family shall have occasion to make use of" during their natural lives, in exchange for 100 acres of land.[23]

The vestry of Christ Church in 1699 agreed with Dr. Robert Deputy "for the Cure of Ellianor Slanter to be paid him when he gives good Security at this County Court for her Cure."[24] Dr. Waldron in 1658 undertook to cure Francis Warren, and "did promise to make hir cure by Xmas or else to have nothing,"[25] and Dr. Rose was to be paid 5,000 pounds of tobacco "provided he make a perfect cure of Jno. Blake a poore Decriped Man of this parish."[26]

21Vestry Book, Christ Church, Middlesex County, p. 38.
22York County Records, v. 6, p. 413.
23Ibid., v. 3, p. 272.
24Vestry Book, Christ Church, Middlesex County, p. 88.
25York County Records, v. 3, p. 107.
26Vestry Book, Christ Church, Middlesex County, p. 10.

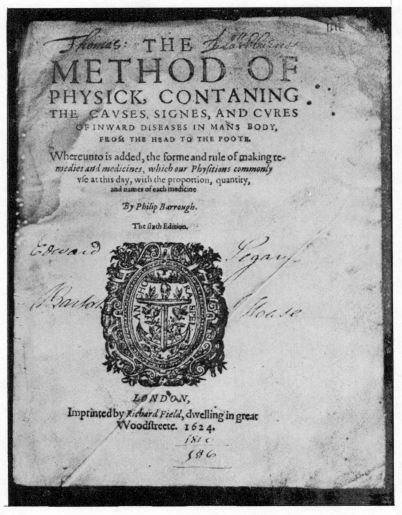

Thomas: THE
METHOD OF
PHYSICK, CONTANING
THE CAVSES, SIGNES, AND CVRES
OF INWARD DISEASES IN MANS BODY,
FROM THE HEAD TO THE FOOTE.

Whereunto is added, the forme and rule of making remedies and medicines, which our Phyſitions commonly
vſe at this day, with the proportion, quantity,
and names of each medicine

By Philip Barrough.

The ſixth Edition.

LONDON,
Imprinted by Richard Field, dwelling in great
Woodſtreete. 1624.

Title page of Barrough's *Method of Physic,* often found in
Seventeenth Century Virginia libraries.

In 1681 John Penny, chirurgeon, made a deposition in York Court that he was sent for to "look upon" Peter Wells, servant of Humphrey Browning, who had been in a fight. Browning asked "what I would have for ye Cure, I told him . . . five pounds, soe he did desire mee to doe it att a reasonable as I could, soe I received three pounds tenn shillings."[27]   In June 1692 John West swore that he heard "Dr. Irby say that he would not exceed fourteen hundred pds of tobo for curing Eliza Mayberry & her daughter of ye Distemper."[28]

A different kind of contract occurs in 1639 in the Northampton County records: "Wee Roger Moye and Anne Moye have and doe by these presents bynde us, ourselves, as servants and to serve dilligently, Wm. Burdett of Accomack or his ass⁵. until that we have ffully satisfied John Stringer of the same County practiconer in Physick ffor a cure that hee hath done upon both our bodyes beinge twelve hundred pounds of good and merchantable tobacco with Caske. . . ."[29]

IV

Collections

From the number of times the physicians appear in court to demand their fees one would infer that collections were

---

[27]York County Records, v. 6, p. 364.
[28]Ibid., v. 5, p. 454.
[29]Northampton County Records, v. 1640-45, p. 28.

not always good. There was a wise Thirteenth Century observation to young physicians: "It is always surer, however, to receive payment while the ailing person is not as yet entirely well, otherwise there is always some risk of not being paid." An unwieldy medium like tobacco rendered impossible a cash and carry policy and made for the accumulation of large bills at the end of a sickness. Often it was necessary to wait until the tobacco crop had been cut and cured and put in the cask.

Typical of the financial difficulties in which the Seventeenth Century doctor often found himself is the case of Dr. Richard Pemberton, whose patient, Thomas Taylor, in 1690 argues in court that his contract was for 500 pounds of tobacco and not the 862 which Dr. Pemberton had charged.[30] Dr. George Eland was frequently in court, appearing twenty-two times to collect his bills. Dr. Henry Power was in court collecting fees seven times between 1680 and 1692.[31] Occasionally the collection of bills led to scenes in court. There is the account of an argument between Dr. John Severne and Mr. Stubbins, each accusing the other of having a certain bill. Dr. Severne "stript himself out of his clothes" to show that he had it not; but Mr. Stubbins replied that "for ought that I know you have throwne it into a hole." Mr. Stubbins then searched himself and found the bill.[32]

[30]Rappahannock County Records, v. 11, p. 226.
[31]York County Records, v. 6, 8, 9.
[32]Northampton County Records, v. 1640-45, p. 197.

In general the Seventeenth Century physician received from thirty-five to fifty pounds of tobacco for a visit. Expressed in modern values, this amounted to between eleven and sixteen dollars. If we assume that he paid only one call a day, his yearly income would have ranged from $4,000 to $6,000.

Chapter XII

MEDICAL LEGISLATION

HE student of Virginia history is indebted to Hening's *Statutes at Large* for much material found nowhere else. Here are collected those early statutes dealing with medical practice in the colony, which, apart from their legal interest, cast a flood of light upon exorbitant medical fees, the cost of medicine, quackery, and the attitude of the public toward the physician of that day.

The first medical practice act to be passed by any of the American colonies was enacted by the Virginia Assembly in 1639. Before the turn of the century seven similar bills had come before the Assembly and been set up by statute. Several of the other colonies were engaged in similar legislation, but not so early.[1]

Many of the acts of the early Virginia Assembly were reproductions of similar English legislation, and many of them were, therefore, anticipative.[2] This is not true of the medical statutes, for there is every evidence that the evils these laws were designed to correct really existed in the colony.

---

[1]Garrison: History of Medicine, p. 308. Packard: History of Medicine in the U. S.
[2]Ingle: Annals of Medical History, v. 5, 1924, p. 248.

The Act of 1639 has been lost, but in 1645 it was re-enacted, probably in identical form, and this bill has been preserved. From it we learn that the colonists were indignant over "the excessive rates and prices exacted by practicioners of physick & chirurgery." Complaints were made to the Assembly that the high cost of medical service kept masters from summoning a doctor for their sick servants, since the cost of a servant's sickness often exceeded his purchase price. The result was that many "hard hearted masters" found it less expensive to let their servants die without medical attention. Under ordinary circumstances masters had a peculiar interest in the health of their servants, and the numerous servant class formed an important part of the physician's practice. In the next century we find a similar interest in the health of the slaves. A planter often sent for a physician to see his slaves when for the same sickness in his own family he would hazard home remedies.

In cases of unreasonable charges the Act of 1645 provided for the arrest of the physician, who was then required to declare the value of the drugs he had prescribed. The decision as to whether or not there had been exorbitant charging was left to the discretion of the court. Where neglect could be shown or it was known that the physician had refused to go to the aid of the sick, the censure of the court was the penalty.

-Act XV of Grand Assembly, March 1645-6:

WHEREAS by the 9th Act of Assembly held the 21st of

October, 1639, consideration being had and taken of the imoderate and excessive rates and prices exacted by practitioners in physick and chyrurgery and the complaints made to the then Assembly of the bad consequence thereof, It so happening through the said intollerable exactions that the hearts of divers masters were hardened rather to suffer their servants to perish for want of fitt meanes and applications then by seeking releife to fall into the hands of griping and avaricious men, It be apprehended by such masters who were more swayed by politick respects then Xpian [Christian] duty or charity, That it was the more gainfull and saving way to stand to the hazard of their servants then to entertain the certain charge of a physitian or chirurgeon whose demands for the most parte exceed the purchase of the patient, It was therefore enacted for the better redress of the like abuses thereafter until some fitter course should be advised on, for the regulating physitians and chirurgeons within the collony, That it should be lawfull and free for any person or persons in such cases where they should conceive the acco't. of the physitian or chirurgeon to be unreasonable either for his pains or for his druggs or medicines, to arrest the said physitian or chirurgeon either to the quarter court or county court where they inhabitt, where the said physitian should declare upon oath the true value worth and quantity of his druggs and medicines administred to or for the use of the plt. whereupon the court where the matter was tryed was to adjudge and allow to the said phisitian or chirurgeon such satisfaction and reward as they in their discretions should think fitt, And it was further ordered that when it should be sufficiently proved in any of the said courts that a physitian or chirurgeon had neglected his patient, or that he had refused, being thereunto required, his helpe and assistance to any person or persons in sicknes or extremity, That the said phisitian or chirurgeon should be censured by the said court for such his neglect or refuseall which said act and every clause therein mentioned and repeated, this present Grand Assembly to all intents and purposes doth revive, rattifie, allow and confirme with this only exception that the plts. or patients shall have their remedie at the county courts respectively, unless in case of appeale.[3]

Evidently the Act was not effective, for it was re-enacted for the third and fourth times.

Act XXXVII of Asembly, March 1657-8:

"For the regulateing of the imoderate excessive rates and prices exacted by practitioners of phisick and chirurgery, Bee it enacted that it shall be lawfull and free for any person or persons where they shall conceive the account of the phisitian or chirurgeon to be unreasonable either for his paines, druggs or medecines to arrest the said phisitian or chirurgeon either to the quarter court or county court where they inhabit, where the said phisitian shall declare upon oath the true valew, worth and quantity of his druggs and medecines administred to or for the use of the plaintiffe, Whereupon the court where the matter is tried shall adjudge and allow the said phisitian or chirurgeon such satisfaction and reward as they in their discretions shall think fitt, And it is further ordered that where it shall be sufficiently proved in any of the said courts that a phisitian or chirurgeon hath neglected his patient, or that he hath refused (being there-

---

[3]Hening: Statutes at Large, v. 1, p. 316.

unto required) his helpe and assistance to any person or persons in sicknes or extremitie, that the said phisitian or chirurgeon shall be censured by the court for such his neglect or refusall."[4]

At the same time the Assembly passed another act, this time favorable to the physicians. It was provided that in case the patient died the physician's fees were collectable out of the estate. Judging by the number of times physicians appear in the court records doing this very thing, this statute must have been a Godsend. One suspects that politics entered largely into the medical legislation of colonial Virginia.

Act XXIV of Assembly, March 1660-1:

WHEREAS by a former act of assembly no accompts are pleadable against dead mens estates whereby some scruples have beene made about the accompts of physitians and Chyrurgeon cannot possibly take bills, Bee itt therefore enacted that physitians and chyrurgeons accompts shall be pleadable and recoverable for meanes administred and paines taken in the fitt of sicknesse whereof the patient dyes, and where the patient recovers six months after such recovery and noe longer.[5]

The next Act, 1661, though much like those preceding it, is also a sad commentary on the practice of medicine. It shows that high fees had continued in spite of legislation, that the grade of medical service given was not thought to

[4]Hening: Statutes at Large, v. 1, p. 450.
[5]Ibid., v. 2, p. 26.

be commensurate with the fees, that charlatans were numerous, and that the public had little respect for the physician. The very wording of the bill is worth noting. The phrase in former bills, that masters "suffer their servants to perish," is now changed to "exposing servants to a hazzard of recovery," and whereas the earlier physicians were spoken of as "griping and avaricious men," the doctor is now called "a rigorous though unskilful physician." Mention is made of "the poore people also" who have to choose between "lingering disease" and "ruine by endeavoring to procure an uncertain remedy."

It was a century of quacks in England, and London boasted many famous ones. There was Arthur Dee, who was brought before the Censors of the College of Physicians. John Lambe was "a bold charlaton, who was charged with demanding forty to fifty pounds for his cures of a Mr. Pickering in Cheapside, who died in his hands." There was a plausible rogue named Thomas Safford, who practised what he called "Christian Astrology." There was also John Case, over whose door was inscribed:

"Within this place
Lives Doctor Case."

Addison said this couplet had made more money for Dr. Case than Dryden had made by all his verse. On a merry evening this same Dr. Case was encountered by the distinguished Dr. Radcliffe, who offered this toast to the quack: "Here's to all the fools, your patients Brother Case!" to which Case replied, "Let me have all the fools, and you are welcome to all the rest of the practice."

There were probably mountebanks in the colony also, though most of the fault lay in poor medical education and blind ignorance on the part of the doctors, rather than in malice. The doctors undoubtedly made extravagant claims for themselves. The very bargaining in which they were constantly engaged with their patients as to the time it would take to effect cures shows that many did not scruple to boast of what they could do; and boasting and quackery are familiar bed-fellows. A century later we find Theodorick Bland, a young medical student, thundering vehemently against the quacks, but there is little evidence that organized quackery was common in Seventeenth Century Virginia, or that there were here any of those professional rogues and rascals who were often popular in England. It is true there was a chirurgeon, John Stringer, who styled himself "Philomedici," but this may have been only an innocent piece of bombast.

Act XCII of Assembly, March 1661-2:

WHEREAS the excessive and immoderate prices exacted by diverse avaritious and gripeing practitioners in phisick and chirurgery hath caused several hardhearted masters swayed by profitable rather then charitiable respects, rather to expose a sick servant to a hazard of recovery, than put themselves to the certaine charge of a rigorous though unskilfull phisician, whose demands for the most part exceed the purchase of the patient, many other poore people also being forced to give themselves over to a lingring disease, rather then ruine themselves by endeavouring to procure an uncertaine remedy, for redrese thereof for the future, Be it enacted that it shalbe lawfull for any person or persons conceiving the accompt of the phisitian or chirurgion unreasonable to arrest the said phisician or chirurgion to the generall or county court where the said phisitian or chirurgion shall declare upon his oath the true value, cost, and quantity of the drugs administred, for which the court shall grant order against the plaintiff with fifty per cent advance, and such consideration for his care, visitts and attendance as they shall judge he hath deserved, and if it shall appeare by evidence that the said phisitian or chirurgion hath neglected his patient while he was under cure, the court shall censure him to pay soe much as they in their discretion shall think reasonable.[6]

By the end of the century there is evidence of the increasing influence of the medical profession in the passage of legislation which again makes physicians' accounts pleadable after the death of the patient and in the revocation of a former act which made them liable to arrest for over charging.

Act XCV of Assembly, March 1661-2:

WHEREAS too sad experience hath shewed that accounts against the estates of persons deceased have often unjustly devowred the estates . . . Bee it therefore enacted that noe booke debts or accompts shalbe henceforth pleadable, in any court of justice in this country, against a dead mans

---

[6]Hening: Statutes at Large, v. 2, p. 109.

estate . . . unless they be such accompts as by particular acts of assembly, as officers fees, levyes, chirurgions accompts are pleadable. . . .[7]

Act IIII of Assembly, April 1692:

Whereas it is expressed and declared in the 92 act of assembly entituled Chyrurgeons accounts regulated, that it shall be lawfull for any person or persons conceiving the accounts of Physician or Chyrurgeon unreasonable, to arrest the said Physician or Chyrurgeon to the generall or county court,

Be it enacted by their Majesties Lieutenant Governour, Councell and Burgesses of this present General Assembly and the authority thereof, and it is hereby enacted, That the same clause be henceforth repealed, and it is hereby repealed, the same being in itselfe unreasonable.

And be it enacted by the authority aforesaid, and it is hereby enacted, That every Physician or Chirurgeon be allowed the true vallue of his druggs and means, with cent per cent upon the first cost, he making oath to the same, and that where the Physician and Chyrurgeon cannot declare upon his oath the first cost of his medicines the court wherein any controversey shall depend about the same, shall and are hereby empowered to give judgment therein according to the best of their knowledge, allowing the physician or chyrurgeon for his care, visitts, and attendance, a recompence suitable to his deserts.[8]

"An act declaring how long judgments, bonds, obligations, and accounts, shall be in force, for the assignment of bonds and obligations, directing what proof shall be suf-

---

[7]Hening: Statutes at Large, v. 2, p. 111.
[8]Ibid., v. 3, p. 103.

ficient in such cases; and ascertaining the damage upon protested bills of exchange," passed in 1705, provided:

". . . . . That when any suit shall be commenced upon a physitians or chirurgeons account it shall be lawfull for the court to put such a reasonable valuation upon the medicines administred, and the visits, attendance and other services performed, as to them shall seem meet and just, any thing herein before contained, to the contrary notwithstanding."[9]

---

[9]Hening: Statutes at Large, v. 3, p. 379.

A BRIEF BIOGRAPHICAL DICTIONARY OF 17TH CENTURY VIRGINIA PHYSICIANS*

ABRAM, DR. THOMAS:
Mentioned in 1700, 1701.
(York Co. Records.)

ADDAMS, DR. WILLIAM:
Northumberland Co. Mentioned in 1654.
(Va. Mag. of Hist. & Biog., v. 1.)

ALLEN, DR. NATHANIELL:
Rappahannock Co. Died 1687.
(Rappahannock Co. Records.)

ALLIN, DR. ————:
Mentioned in 1673.
(Surry Co. Records.)

ANDREWS, DR. HENRY:
York Co. First mentioned 1693. Died Nov. 1705.
(York & Surry Co. Records; Wm. & Mary Quart., v. 2.)

ARNOLD, DR. ————:
Mentioned 1686.
(Rappahannock Co. Records.)

AYLETT, MR. THOMAS:
Probably a chirurgeon. Mentioned 1678-1690.
(York & Henrico Co. Records.)

---

*The title "Doctor," is used wherever the men were so called in the records, and does not necessarily mean that they had the M. D. degree. When they were called "chirurgeon" in the records, that title is given them.

BAGNALL, ANTHONY:
Chirurgeon. Came to Va. in 1607 or 1608, and accompanied Smith on his second expedition up Chesapeake Bay.
(Smith: General History.)

BANISTER, REV. JOHN:
Naturalist. Graduate of Oxford. Lived in Charles City Co., Va., from 1678 to his death in 1692. His catalogue of Va. plants was published in Ray's *Historia Plantarum*. Other scientific writings were: *Insects of Virginia, Curiosities in Virginia, On Several Sorts of Snails, Description of the Snake Root*. He was a minister of the Church of England.
(Va. Mag. of Hist. & Biog., v. 11; Goodwin: Colonial Church; Philos. Trans. Royal Soc.)

BANKES, DR. WILLIAM:
Listed among civil officers of Stafford Co., 1680. Recommended by Wm. Fitzhugh for High Sheriff, 1682.
(Va. Mag. of Hist. & Biog., v. 1: Fitzhugh Letters.)

BANTON, DR. ————:
Mentioned, 1672.
(Surry Co. Records.)

BAYLEY, GEORGE:
Chirurgeon, of Plymouth, Eng. Purchased 300 acres in Va. in 1671.
(Rappahannock Co. Records.)

BELFIELD, DR. JOSEPH:
Emigrated from England to Richmond Co., Va., before 1707. Died in Va. in 1738.

(Va. Mag. of Hist. & Biog., v. 24; Hayden: Va. Genealogies, p. 13.)

BILL, DR. ROBERT:
Mentioned, 1701.
(York Co. Records.)

BLAGRAVE, HENRY:
Practised in York Co., 1661-1668.
(York Co. Records.)

BLAKE, THOMAS:
Chirurgeon, James City Co., 1693.
(York Co. Records.)

BOCOCKE, DR. ————:
Practised in Eliz. City Co., 1690.
(Eliz. City Co. Records.)

BOHUN (BOHUNE), DR. LAWRENCE:
Studied medicine in the Netherlands. Came to Va. with Lord Delaware in 1610 and returned with him to England. Appointed Physician-General of Va., Dec. 1620. On his way to the colony, in March 1621, he was killed in a seafight with two Spanish Men of War.
(Records of Va. Co.)

BONMAN, DR. ————:
Physician to Thomas Jefferson, ancestor of President Jefferson, in 1698.
(Va. Mag. of Hist. & Biog., v. 1.)

BOODLE, DR. ROBERT:
Middlesex Co. Married in 1685. Employed by Christ Church Vestry to treat poor of the Parish, 1683.

(Parish Register & Vestry Book, Christ Church, Middlesex Co.)

BOOTH, DR. ROBERT:
York Co.   His daughter married Dr. Patrick Napier.
(Va. Mag. of Hist. & Biog., v. 33, p. 45.)

BOWMAN, DR. JOHN:
Practised in Henrico Co., 1689-97.   Presented to the Grand Jury in 1692 "for swearing 2 oaths."
(Henrico Co. Records.)

BOWMAN, SIMON:
Chirurgeon.   Practised in 1640.
(Minutes of Council & General Court.)

BRASEY (BEASEY), DR. WILLIAM:
Practised in 1686-87.
(Rappahannock Co. Records.)

BROCK, JOHN:
Chirurgeon.   Owned land in York Co. in 1647.
(York Co. Records.)

BUNN, THOMAS:
Chirurgeon.   Practised 1624-26.
(Minutes of Council & General Court.)

BURGANY, DR. ————:
Mentioned, 1672.
(Minutes of Council & Gen. Court.)

BURN, THOMAS:
Ship Surgeon on the *Young Prince,* sent to Va. during Bacon's Rebellion, 1676.
(Calendar British State Papers.)

CAGAN, DR. ————— :
>   Practised in 1678.
>   (Henrico Co. Records.)

CHAPPELL, DR. ALEXANDER:
>   Practised in 1693-94.
>   (Richmond Co. Records.)

CHERMESON (CHERMISON), DR. JOSEPH:
>   Practised in Bruton Parish, York Co., 1688-1702, and
>   was apparently prosperous.
>   (York Co. Records.)

CHERRICHOLM, MARMADUKE:
>   Chirurgeon. Son of an apothecary in England. His
>   will proved in Isle of Wight Co. in 1690. He moved
>   to New England before his death.
>   (Wm. & Mary Quart., v. 7.)

CLARK, DR. ROBERT:
>   Practised in Rappahannock Co., 1685-90, and Rich-
>   mond Co. 1694.
>   (Rappahannock & Richmond Co. Records.)

CLAY, CHARLES:
>   Apprenticed in 1657 for seven years to Stephen Tick-
>   ner to learn "Chyrurgerye, or Phissicke."
>   (Surry Co. Records.)

CLAYTON, REV. JOHN:
>   Church of England clergyman, Fellow Royal Society,
>   and naturalist. Was Minister at Jamestown, 1684-
>   86, and also seems to have practised medicine. Wrote
>   an *Account of Virginia* for the Royal Society, contain-
>   ing many scientific observations.
>   (Force: Tracts; Philos. Trans., Royal Soc.)

CLEVERIUS, JOHN:
Chirurgeon. Died about 1657.
(York Co. Records.)

CLOPTON, ISAAC:
Practised in York Co. Justice of the Peace from 1675 until his death in 1677/8.
(York Co. Records.)

CLOYBURNE, ————:
Chirurgeon. Came over in 1621 with Gov. Wyatt and Dr. Pott.
(Smith: General History.)

CLULO, DR. JOHN:
Practised in 1658.
(York Co. Records.)

COGAN, JOHN:
Chirurgeon, of Jordans Parish, Charles City Co., 1656.
(Surry Co. Records.)

COOPER, CHRISTOPHER:
Chirurgeon. Mentioned, 1671.
(Rappahannock Co. Records.)

CORDON, DR. ————:
Lower Norfolk Co. Mentioned, 1656.
(Bruce: Institutional History of Va.)

CRIMES, DR. WILLIAM:
Mentioned, 1697-99, in York Co. A "William Crimes of Glocester County Gent." bought 500 acres in Rappahannock Co. in 1686.
(York & Rappahannock Co. Records.)

CULMER, THOMAS:
Chirurgeon, of Lawnes Creek Parish, Surry Co.,
1655-62.   Owned land and practised law as well as
medicine.
(Surry Co. Records.)

CURLEEN, RICHARD:
Administered physic to the servants of Col. Daniel
Parke in 1679.
(York Co. Records.)

DANZE (DANZEE), DR. JOHN JACOB COIGNAN:
Practised in York Co., 1688-98.
(York Co. Records.)

DAVIS, DR. EDWARD:
Practised in Surry Co., 1652.
(Surry Co. Records.)

DAVIS, GEORGE:
"Phisitian," of Rappahannock Co.   Practised law and
medicine, 1664-67.
(Rappahannock Co. Records.)

DENT, ANTHONY:
Practised in 1686.
(York Co. Records.)

DEPUTIE (DEPUTY), DR. ROBERT:
Chirurgeon.   Married Anne Wright, Feb. 23, 1679,
and Mary Huddle, Oct. 9, 1707, in Christ Church
Parish, Middlesex Co.   Employed by Christ Church
Vestry in 1699.   Owned 200 acres in Rappahannock
Co. in 1690.
(Parish Register & Vestry Book, Christ Church, Mid-
dlesex Co.; Rappahannock Co. Records.)

DIXON, DR. —————:
Mentioned, 1667.
(York Co. Records.)

DUNAVANT, PETER:
Chirurgeon. Mentioned, 1671.
(Rappahannock Co. Records.)

DUNNING, RICHARD:
Administered physic in 1648. Churchwarden of New
Poquoson Parish, York Co.
(York Co. Records.)

EATON, THOMAS:
Physician. Lived in Va. a number of years and
founded the Eaton Free School on land patented by
him in Eliz. City Co. in 1634.
(Bruce: Institutional History of Va.)

EDWARDS, JOHN:
Chirurgeon, Lancaster Co. Sold some land in 1653.
Died March 1667, and bequeathed land, servants,
personal property, and a share in the Ship *Susan*.
(Va. Mag. of Hist. & Biog., v. 5; Wm. & Mary
Quart., v. 20.)

EEDES, ROBERT:
Ship Surgeon, 1627.
(Minutes of Council & General Court.)

ELAND, DR. GEORGE:
Mentioned frequently in Eliz. City Co., 1688-97, as
physician, executor of estates, etc. In 1697 he was
appointed master of the Eaton School.
(Eliz. City Co. Records; Bruce: Institutional History
of Va.)

ELLIS, DR. WILLLIAM:
Practised in York & Eliz. City Co.   Died 1698.
(York & Eliz. City Co. Records.)

ELLYSON, DR. ROBERT:
Mentioned as "barber-chirurgeon" in Maryland, 1643.
First mentioned in Va. in 1649, as "Chyrurgion" in
Surry Co.   Was High Sheriff and Coroner of James
City Co. in 1657; member House of Burgesses, 1656,
1659-60, 1660-61, 1663.   Referred to as "Captain"
and "Doctor" in York Co., where he was active as
physician, attorney and public official.   Died about
1671.
(Surry & York Co. Records; Minutes of Council &
General Court; Wm. & Mary Quart., v. 6.)

FIELD, THOMAS:
Apothecary.   Came to Va. with the first supply, 1608.
(Smith: General History.)

FITCH, JOSEPH:
Apothecary to Dr. Pott.   Massacred by the Indians in
March, 1622.
(Neill: Va. Co. of London.)

GERARD (GERRARD), THOMAS:
Physician.   Was a Privy Councillor in Maryland, but
in 1658 was tried on charges of intemperance and op-
position to Lord Baltimore, and deposed from the
Council.   Settled in Westmoreland Co., Va., where he
became a prominent and wealthy citizen.   His will was
proved Nov. 19, 1673.
(Encyc. Va. Biog.; Neill: Va. Carolorum.)

GIBSON, DR. ————— :

His plantation in Rappahannock Co. mentioned in a deed, 1671.

(Rappahannock Co. Records.)

GIBSON, ED.:

Mentioned in Minutes of Council & General Court as having before 1622 cured a number of persons at the settlement at Falling Creek.

(Va. Mag. of Hist. & Biog., v. 19.)

GILL, CAPTAIN STEPHEN G.:

Chirurgeon. Patented land in York Co. in 1638. Active in the practice of medicine. A Justice of York Co. and Burgess in 1652. Apparently could not sign his name. Died in 1653, leaving a rather large estate.

(York Co. Records; Va. Mag. of Hist. & Biog., v. 6.)

GINNAT, POST:

Chirurgeon. Came to Va. with the first supply in 1608.

(Smith: General History.)

GLOVER, THOMAS:

Chirurgeon. Wrote an *Account of Virginia*, published in the Philos. Trans. of the Royal Soc., 1676.

GREEN, DR. ————— :

Nathaniel Bacon said to have died at his house in Gloucester County, 1676. This is probably an error.

(Oldmixon, British Empire.)

GREEN, WILLIAM:

Ship Surgeon, 1623-28.

(Minutes of Council & General Court.)

GREENWOOD, GERRARD:
Administered "phisicall meanes" in Rappahannock Co. in 1687.
(Rappahannock Co. Records.)

GREINE, DR. ————:
Mentioned in a will, 1683. He may be the same as Dr. Green, above, mentioned by Oldmixon.
(Rappahannock Co. Records.)

GROVER, JONATHAN:
Surgeon of the expedition sent to Va. from England, following Bacon's Rebellion, 1676.
(Calendar British State Papers.)

GUNNELL, GEORGE:
Chirurgeon. Mentioned as absconding to Maryland, leaving unpaid debts, in 1689.
(Eliz. City Co. Records.)

GWYN, DR. EDWARD:
Gloucester Co. Mentioned, 1678, 1683. Referred to in a genealogy of the Gwyn (Gwin) family as "a regular Doctor of Physick," son of Rev. John Gwin of Abingdon Parish, who came to Va. in Cromwell's time.
(Executive Journals, Council of Colonial Va.; Va. Mag. of Hist. & Biog., v. 4, p. 204.)

HACKE, DR. GEORGE:
Born in Cologne, Germany, about 1623. Received a grant of 400 acres in Northampton Co., Va., in 1653, and also owned land in Northumberland Co. Was a leading practitioner in Northampton Co. Naturalized

at the 1658 session of the Grand Assembly. Died,
1666. His son, Peter, was Burgess from Northumberland in 1706, and Colonel of Militia; and his other
son, George Nicholas, was Sheriff of Accomack Co.
in 1700.
(Journals House of Burgesses; Executive Journals,
Council of Colonial Va.; Va. Mag. of Hist. & Biog.)

HADDON, DR. FRANCIS:
Came to Va. under terms of indenture about 1656.
In 1658 married the widow of Dr. Giles Modé. Had
a large practice in York Co. and was often in court
to collect bills for "phisick and attendance." Died in
1674, leaving a fairly large estate.
(York Co. Records.)

HAINESWORTH, DR. ————:
Mentioned, 1678.
(Surry Co. Records.)

HALL, DR. RICHARD:
Mentioned in 1643 as "practiconer in phisick." In
1652 he received land grants for the importation of six
members of his family.
(Northampton Co. Records; Greer: Early Va. Immigrants.)

HALLOM (HALLUM), DR. ————:
Mentioned in 1671, 1675. Died about 1679.
(York Co. Records.)

HARFORD, THOMAS:
Apothecary. Came to Va. in 1608 with the first supply.
(Smith: General History.)

HARRILD (HAVEILD), DR. LUKE:
Was granted land in Nansemond Co., 1694. Mentioned, 1705.
(Executive Journals, Council of Colonial Va.; Wm. & Mary Quart., v. 7.)

HARRIS, EDWARD:
Chirurgeon. One of the medical attendants of Col. Daniel Parke and an appraiser of Col. Parke's estate, 1679.
(York Co. Records.)

HARRIS, DR. JOHN:
Lancaster Co., 1683.
(Bruce: Institutional History of Va.)

HARRISON, DR. JEREMY (JEREMIAH):
His passage to Va. was paid for in 1654 by "Mrs. Fra: Harrison, widow." He is said to have been a Cavalier immigrant. His wife, Frances, was daughter of Thomas Whitgreave, who saved the life of Charles II at Worcester. Dr. Harrison patented land in York Co. He is probably the same as the "Dr. Harrison" mentioned in Surry Co. in 1655. Deceased before 1672, when his land was granted to the parish of Middletowne.
(Greer: Early Va. Immigrants; Surry Co. Records; Minutes of Council & General Court; Wm. & Mary Quart., v. 6.)

HAY, DR. JOHN:
Said to have come to Va. in 1696 from England, where he was known as "John Gray." Justice of Middlesex Co. in 1706, and died in 1709.

(Calendar Va. State Papers; Va. Mag. of Hist. & Biog., v. 3.)

HELDER, EDMOND:
According to his tombstone, found on Potomac Creek, Stafford Co., Va., he was "practioner in Physick and Chyrurgery," born in Bedfordshire, England, died March 11, 1618, aged 76.
(Harpers Magazine, Jan. 1886.)

HENRY, DR. JOHN:
Middlesex Co. Left a large library.
(Va. Mag. of Hist. & Biog., v. 3.)

HEWES, RICHARD:
Ship Surgeon, 1626.
(Minutes of Council & General Court.)

HILL, NATHANIEL:
Schoolmaster. Probably also had medical training, as his inventory includes a number of medical books and instruments. Moved from Gloucester to Henrico Co. in 1686, and died 1687.
(Henrico Co. Records.)

HITCH, HENRY:
Ship Surgeon, 1623.
(Neill: Va. Co. of London.)

HOLLOWAY, DR. JOHN:
A leading physician of Accomac Co. from 1633 until his death in 1643. Left a rather large estate, including land and servants. Frequently involved in litigation. Arrested for blasphemy and adultery, but seems

to have been well thought of, and was on friendly terms with the minister of his parish.
(Northampton Co. Records.)

HOPEGOOD, PETER:
Chirurgeon. Born 1647, probably in England. Practised in 1677-79, dying in the latter year. Left an estate in England.
(Rappahannock Co. Records.)

HOPKINS, GEORGE:
Chirurgeon. Died 1644.
(York Co. Records.)

HUBBART, DR. MOSES:
Had a large practice in Rappahannock and Richmond Co., 1684-92.
(Rappahannock & Richmond Co. Records.)

HUSLESCOTT, THOMAS:
Administered physic in Rappahannock Co. in 1686.
(Rappahannock Co. Records.)

IKEN (IKIN), DR. THOMAS:
Sheriff of Warwick Co. in 1670. Mentioned as practising in York Co., 1667-70.
(York Co. Records.)

INMAN, JOHN:
Surgeon. Came to Va. as a servant before 1628. "John Iniman" is one of the living in "Lists of the Livinge & Dead in Virginia, Feb. 1623."
(Minutes of Council & Gen. Court.)

INNIS, WALTER:
Chirurgeon. Mentioned in 1689, 1693.
(Eliz. City Co. Records.)

IRBY, DR. WILLIAM:
Lived in Westover Parish, Charles City Co., and
owned land there. Collected medical fees in Henrico
Co. Court, 1679-1693. Went to England in 1693,
but was back in 1695.
(Henrico Co. Records; Carrington: Halifax Co.)

IRONMONGER, DR. ————:
Mentioned, 1681.
(Surry Co. Records.)

JACKSON, DR. MATTHEW:
Mentioned in Stafford Co., 1700.
(Va. Mag. of Hist. & Biog., v. 18.)

JACOB, ————:
Ship surgeon, 1679.
(York Co. Records.)

JANSON, DR. GEORGE:
Gloucester Co., mentioned in 1698.
(Eliz. City & York Co. Records, v. 11.)

JOHNSON, DR. ROBERT:
Of York River. Mentioned as doctor and "Chy-
rurgion" in 1670, 1671.
(York Co. Records.)

JONES, MAURICE:
Ship Surgeon. Died in 1658.
(York Co. Records.)

JONES, DR. WALTER:
Practised in 1684-99.
(Eliz. City Co. Records.)

JUICE, DR. NATHANIEL:
Practised in Christ Church Parish, Middlesex Co., in 1704, 1706.
(Vestry book, Christ Church.)

JULIAN, JOHN:
Chirurgeon, stationed at Potomac Garrison, 1682.
(Journals House of Burgesses.)

KENTON, HENRY:
Chirurgeon. Killed by Indians on the Eastern Shore, 1603, while on an expedition under Capt. Bartholomew Gilbert.
(Brown: Genesis.)

KIPPINGE, ANDREW:
Chirurgeon. Mentioned, 1648.
(Surry Co. Records.)

KNIGHT, JOHN:
Surgeon-General of the Expedition to Va. following Bacon's Rebellion, 1676.
(Calendar British State Papers.)

KNIGHT, DR. NATHANIEL:
Owned a plantation in Southwarke Parish, Surry Co., and practised there between 1663 and his death in 1677.
(Surry Co. Records.)

LEDERER, DR. JOHN:
German surgeon, sent by Gov. Berkeley on three expeditions of discovery into Western Virginia, 1669-70. He wrote *The Discoveries of John Lederer in Three Several Marches from Virginia,* published in London,

1672. A "Doctor Liderer," who practised in Surry Co. in 1672, may have been the same person.
(Lederer: Discoveries, etc.; Glover: Account of Va.; Groome: Fauquier Co.; Surry Co. Records.)

LEE, DR. GEORGE:
Practised in Surry Co. from 1673 or earlier, until 1680, when he was granted a lease of two houses and fifty acres at Jamestown. Was frequently paid by the County for providing lodgings for soldiers, burgesses, etc., and apparently had a large medical practice.
(Surry Co. Records; Henrico Co. Records; Journals House of Burgesses.)

LEE, DR. HENRY, SR.:
Practised in York Co., 1646. Burgess from Northumberland Co., 1651-52. Justice of York Co., 1653. Died 1657, leaving fairly large estate.
(York Co. Records; Journals House of Burgesses.)

LEE, DR. JOHN:
Eldest son of Col. Richard Lee. Was at Oxford before 1658, and later took his M. D. somewhere in England. Died in Va. in 1674.
(Bruce: Institutional History of Va.; Wm. & Mary Quart., v. 6.)

LEVETT, THOMAS:
Ship Surgeon. Mentioned, 1679.
(York Co. Records.)

LOMAX, DR. JOHN:
Married Elizabeth, daughter of Col. Ralph Wormeley. Practised in Christ Church Parish, Middlesex

Co., in 1701. Owned land in Essex Co., 1704, and was Justice in 1706.
(Executive Journals, Council of Colonial Va.; Vestry Book, Christ Church; Wm. & Mary Quart., v. 17.)

Love, James:
Probably a ship surgeon. Died 1681.
(Rappahannock Co. Records.)

Luellin, Henry:
Chirurgeon-General of an expedition against the Indians in 1644.
(Va. Mag. of Hist. & Biog., v. 23.)

Madox, William:
Chirurgeon, of Hampton Parish, York Co., 1669.
(York Co. Records.)

Makemie, Francis:
"Father of the Presbyterian Church in America," was said to have been a doctor of physic as well as a minister. Came to Accomac Co., Va., soon after 1684, and died there in 1708.
(Executive Journals, Council of Colonial Va.; Wise: Eastern Shore.)

Meckeny, Alexander:
Mentioned as practising medicine, 1694.
(Henrico Co. Records.)

Micou, Dr. Paul:
Born 1658; died 1736. Mentioned as practising medicine in Richmond Co., 1693, 1694.
(Richmond Co. Records; Notes on Culpeper Co.)

MODÉ (MOODY), DR. GILES:
Probably a Frenchman. Was naturalized in Va. in 1655, and Justice of York Co. the same year. Practised medicine in York Co. and died there in 1657, leaving land, house, servants and considerable personal property. Had three sons, Josias, Humphrey and Philip.
(York Co. Records; Va. Historical Collections, v. 11; Journals House of Burgesses.)

MOLE, SAMUEL:
Chirurgeon. Was in Va. 1620-23.
(Neill: Va. Co. of London.)

MONTGOMERY, DR. JAMES:
Surgeon of the man-of-war, *St. Albans*. Died in England about 1697, leaving property in Va.
(Bruce: Social Life in Va.)

MONTONE, DR. JOHN:
A Frenchman, came to Va. about 1643 and settled in Northumberland Co. Petitioned for naturalization in 1663. Was probably a Huguenot.
(Northumberland Co. Order Book, 1663.)

MOORE, DR. ————:
Mentioned, 1667.
(York Co. Records.)

NAPIER, DR. PATRICK:
Came to Va. about 1655 and settled in Hampton Parish, York Co., where he had a large practice. Died in 1669, leaving 1,500 acres in New Kent Co. to his wife, Elizabeth.
(York Co. Records.)

NAPIER, VALENTINE:
   "Phisitian," of New Kent Co.   Brother of Dr. Patrick
   Napier.   Mentioned in 1668, 1679.
   (York Co. Records.)

NORTON, CAPT. WILLIAM:
   Said by Capt. John Smith to have been a physician,
   killed in the Indian Massacre, 1622.   He may have
   been the same as Capt. William Norton who brought
   over a group of Italians to start a glass-works in 1623
   and died soon after.
   (Smith: General History; Records of the Va. Co.)

OASTLER, DR. WILLIAM:
   Employed by Vestry of Christ Church for medical
   services, 1697.
   (Vestry Book, Christ Church, Middlesex Co.)

OSBURNE, DR. ————:
   Mentioned, 1687.
   (Rappahannock Co. Records.)

OVERSTREETE, JOHN:
   Mentioned as practising medicine in York Co. between
   1659 and 1670.   Received 250 acres in 1666, for transportation of five persons.   His will probated in Oct.
   1671.
   (York Co. Records.)

PARKE (PARK), COLONEL DANIEL:
   Born in England about 1628 and came to Va. very
   young.   Justice of York Co. for many years, beginning
   1653.   Sheriff of York Co. 1659, and again in 1665.
   Burgess in 1666-68; member of the Council, 1670;

Secretary of State and Treasurer of the Colony, 1678-79. Married Rebecca, daughter of George Evelyn. Died March 6, 1679, and is buried in Bruton Parish Church, Williamsburg. He was an active practising physician, as well as a merchant, lawyer and planter, and frequently collected bills for medical services in York Co. Court between 1658 and 1674. He was a very large landowner. His will, filed in London, bequeathes "all my Plantations and negroes in Virginia" and most of his estate "in Virginia and England" to his son, Daniel Parke, who had a colorful career as member of parliament, aide to the Duke of Marlborough at Blenheim, and Governor of the Leeward Islands, where he was murdered in a riot in 1710. The younger Daniel Parke had a daughter, Lucy, who was the first wife of William Byrd II, of Westover.

(York Co. Records; Va. Mag. of Hist. & Biog., v. 14.)

PARKER, DR. DAVID:
Lived in Prince George Co. His will probated in 1717.
(Va. Mag. of Hist. & Biog., v. 7.)

PARKER, DR. RICHARD:
Born in England. Received grants of land in Northampton, Nansemond, Henrico and Surry Counties, Va., at various times between 1654 and 1676.
(Henrico Co. Records; Va. Mag. of Hist. & Biog., v. 5.)

PATE, DR. (JOHN):
Nathaniel Bacon, the Rebel, was said to have died at the house of a Dr. Pate, in Gloucester Co. in 1676.

There was a John Pate in Goucester at this time, who
was member of the Council in 1670 and died in 1681.
His nephew, Thomas Pate, was Justice of Gloucester
in 1680.   Bacon probably died at the house of one of
them.

(Campbell: History of Va.; Va. Mag. of Hist. &
Biog., v. 4.)

PAWLETT, REV. ROBERT:

Came to Va. in 1619 as preacher, surgeon and physician.   Lived at Martin's Hundred.   Was appointed
to the Council in 1621, but declined to serve.

(Records of the Va. Co.; Neill: Va. Vetusta.)

PAWLEY, JOHN:

Chirurgeon.   Patented 500 acres in James City Co.,
July 20, 1639.

(Abstracts of Patents, Land Office, James City Book I,
p. 661.)

PAYNE, DR. ————:

Mentioned in 1689.

(Executive Journals, Council of Colonial Va.)

PEMBERTON, DR. RICHARD:

Practised medicine, 1684-90.

(Rappahannock Co. Records.)

PENNY, JOHN:

Chirurgeon.   Practising in 1681.

(York Co. Records.)

PETEET (PETIT, PETEETE), JOHN:

Chirurgeon.   A Frenchman, born about 1611.   Settled
in York Co., where he owned land and practised medi-

cine between 1657 and 1670. Was naturalized in
1666. His will was filed April 26, 1670.
(York Co. Records.)

PHILLIPS, DR. WILLIAM:
Mentioned, 1674, 1679.
(York Co. Records; Minutes of Council & General
Court.)

PLOVIER (PLUVIER, PLUVIERE, PLOVER), PETER:
Chirurgeon. Probably a Frenchman. Practised medi-
cine in Warwick Co. in 1659, but in 1666 had moved
to Poquoson Parish, York Co., where he owned land.
Died, 1677/8.
(York Co. Records.)

PLOWRIGHT, SAMUELL:
Chirurgeon. Lived in York Co. in 1668, but was in
London in 1670, and in Va. again in 1675.
(York Co. Records.)

POND, DR. SAMUEL:
Practised in York Co., 1680-94. According to his
tombstone at Martin's Hundred, he lived in James
City Co. and died there Oct. 26, 1694, aged 48.
(Va. Historical Collections, v. 11.)

POOLE, HENRY:
Chirurgeon of Elizabeth City Co. Burgess in 1647-48.
(York Co. Records, v. 3; Journals House of Bur-
gesses.)

POOLE, DR. WILLIAM:
Middlesex Co. Paid by Christ Church Vestry for
medical services, 1678-85. Died Feb. 29, 1687.
(Parish Register & Vestry Book, Christ Church.)

POTT (POTTS), DR. JOHN:

Master of Arts, and "Well practised in Chirurgerie and Phisique," accepted the position of Physician-General to Va. in July 1621. Member of the Council, but lost his seat in 1624 because he was thought to have been responsible for poisoning the Indians. Regained his seat in 1626, and became temporary Governor in 1629. In 1630 he was convicted of hog-stealing, but the sentence was suspended, and he was finally pardoned by the King. Was active in political agitations against Gov. John Harvey, his bitter enemy. Died before 1642.
(Records of Va. Co.; Minutes of Council; Brown: First Repub.)

POWELL, DR. MOSES:

Practised in Isle of Wight Co., 1671.
(Wm. & Mary Quart., v. 7.)

POWER, DR. HENRY:

Practising in York Co. in 1680. Married Mary, daughter of Rev. Edward Foliott, of Hampton Parish. Died 1692. He was possibly the same Henry Power who was born in Yorkshire, England, and matriculated at Christ's College, Cambridge, in 1674.
(York Co. Records; Va. Mag. of Hist. & Biog., v. 33.)

PYBUS, DR. JOHN:

Charles City Co. Mentioned as practising also in Henrico Co., 1686-98.
(Henrico Co. Records.)

RAWLINS (RAWLINGS), DR. JEREMIAH:
Practising in York Co., 1658-66.
(York Co. Records.)

REYNOLDS, DR. CORNELIUS:
Owned land in Rappahannock Co. in 1678. Died
about 1685.
(Rappahannock Co. Records.)

REYNOLDS (RENNELLS), DR. THOMAS:
Chirurgeon, of Martin's Brandon, Charles City Co.
Practised in Surry Co. in 1654-65, and bought 100
acres of land there.
(Surry Co. Records.)

RICHARDS, DR. ————:
Mentioned, 1679.
(York Co. Records.)

ROBINS, OBEDIENCE:
Chirurgeon. Born in Northamptonshire, England,
April 16, 1600. Settled in Northampton Co., Va., and
was a Burgess at the sessions of March 1629-30, Jan.
1639, April 1642, Oct. 1644, April 1652 and Nov.
1652. Appointed to the Council in 1655. Died, 1662.
(Minutes of Council & General Court; Va. Mag. of
Hist. & Biog., v. 28.)

ROBINS, DR. THOMAS:
Chirurgeon, of Robins' Neck, Gloucester Co. Mentioned as practising in York Co., 1666-74. In 1666
he married Mary Hansford, whose brother, Thomas,
was executed by Gov. Berkeley in 1676 for supporting
Bacon. He died in 1677.
(York Co. Records; Va. Historical Collections, v. 11.)

ROOTES, DR. THOMAS:
Chirurgeon, of Lancaster Co. His book-plate, pre-
served in a volume in the library of the Richmond
Academy of Medicine (Miller Collection), is in-
scribed: "Doc . . . in Physic Lancaster Coll: of Virgᵃ."
His will is dated Jan. 25, 1660.
(Va. Mag. of Hist. & Biog., v. 5.)

ROSE, DR. ————:
Paid for medical services by Christ Church Vestry,
Middlesex Co., 1667. Probably the same person as
Dr. John Rose, below.
(Vestry Book, Christ Church.)

ROSE, DR. JOHN:
Chirurgeon. Mentioned in 1658-67.
(York Co. Records.)

ROWSLEY, WILLIAM:
Chirurgeon. Received patent for land, July 3, 1622,
and arrived in Virginia in 1623. Died soon afterwards.
(Records Va. Co., v. 2; Neill: Va. Vetusta.)

RUSSELL, MR. ————:
"Acmunist and Chimist." In 1620 he tried unsuccess-
fully to introduce an artificial wine, made of Sassafras
and Licorice, into Va.
(Brown: First Republic.)

RUSSELL, JOHN:
Chirurgeon, of Northumberland Co. Bought 2,250
acres in Rappahannock Co. in 1673, and practised in
that county in 1682.
(Rappahannock Co. Records.)

RUSSELL, DR. RICHARD:

Lived in Lower Norfolk Co. Was interested in raising silkworms in Va., and is the "learned physician"
mentioned in John Ferrar's poem in *The Reformed
Virginian Silk-Worm*, written in 1653, and published
in Force: Tracts, v. 3. Russell later moved to New
England.
(Wm. & Mary Quart., v. 7; Force: Tracts, v. 3.)

RUSSELL, DR. WALTER:

Came to Va. with the First Supply in 1608, and accompanied Capt. Smith on his expedition to explore Chesapeake Bay the same year.
(Smith: General History.)

SAUNDERS (SANDERS), DR. EDWARD:

Mentioned in York Co., 1668. Owned land in Lancaster Co. in 1672. Lived in Northumberland Co. in
1660.
(York & Rappahannock Co. Records.)

SCOTT, ———:

"Phisician." He accompanied Thomas Young on an
expedition to explore the undiscovered parts of Virginia in 1634.
(Calendar British State Papers.)

SEARLE, GABRIEL:

Apprenticed to Dr. John Holloway in 1638 to learn
the art of chirurgery. Was 18 years old in 1643, when
his term of indenture expired.
(Northampton Co. Records.)

SEVERNE, JOHN:

Chirurgeon. Collected numerous fees for medical attendance in Northampton Co., 1638-44. Was granted 300 acres for the transportation of himself and four others, and was apparently a leading citizen in his county. Died in the summer of 1644, leaving a rather small estate.
(Northampton Co. Records.)

SEVERNE, DR. JOHN, JR.:

Son of John Severne, above. Born 1634. Was living in Northampton Co. in 1653.
(Northampton Co. Records; Va. Mag. of Hist. & Biog., v. 19.)

SHEMANS, RAPHAEL:

Ship Surgeon on the *Great Hopewell,* 1636.
(Va. Mag. of Hist. & Biog., v. 13.)

SHREWSBURY, KATHARINE:

Richmond Co. Was a school teacher, and apparently also practised medicine. In 1693 she brought suit to collect a fee for medical attendance.
(Bruce: Institutional History of Va., v. 1.)

SICCARY, DR. ————:

A Portugese physician, said by Thomas Jefferson to have introduced the tomato into Virginia.

SIMONS (SYMMONDS), DR. HUMPHRY:

Mentioned, 1678-79.
(York Co. Records.)

SLADER, DR. MATTHEW:

Practised in York Co., 1672-74. In 1674 he was put in the stocks for cheating in a horse race.
(York Co. Records.)

SMITH, EDMOND:

Chirurgeon. Collected a medical fee in York Co. in 1660. An indentured servant named Edmond Smith, mentioned in 1644, may have been the same person.
(York Co. Records.)

SMITH, DR. RALPH:

In 1687 he married the sister of William Fitzhugh, who describes him in a letter as "an ingenious trader into this Country, a Skilful & Quaint Surgeon . . . and one of considerable Reputation and Substance at Bristol [England] where he lives, but intends this year to transfer his whole concerns hither & here settle . . ." He died before 1692, leaving a large estate to his wife.
(Fitzhugh Letters, in Va. Mag. of Hist. & Biog., v. 2, 4.)

SPEARS, DR. ————:

Practising in 1678.
(Henrico Co. Records.)

SPRUELL, DR. GODFREY:

Owned land and practised medicine in Henrico Co., 1690-95.
(Henrico Co. Records.)

STAPLETON (THOMAS) :
Paid for medical services by vestry of Christ Church,
Middlesex Co., 1684, 1693.
(Vestry Book, Christ Church.)

STARKE (STARK), DR. RICHARD:
Practised in York Co. from 1686 to 1704, when he
died, leaving a large estate. He owned land in both
York and Warwick Counties.
York Co. Records; Va. Mag. of Hist. & Biog., v. 33.)

STONE, DR. JOHN:
Born about 1631. Justice of Rappahannock Co. in
1683 and succeeding years. Sheriff of Rappahannock
in 1691, and of Richmond Co. in 1692. Justice of
Richmond Co., 1693. Was referred to as both Col-
onel and Doctor, and was a large landowner.
(Rappahannock & Richmond Co. Records; Executive
Journals Council of Colonial Va., v. 1; Minutes of
Council & General Court.)

STRINGER, JOHN:
Referred to as "practiconer in Phisick," "Chirurgeon,"
and "philomedici." Practised in Northampton Co.,
1637-43. Member House of Burgesses, 1658-59.
(Northampton Co. Records; Journals House of Burgesses.)

SYNOCK, DR. ROBERT:
Surgeon to Rappahannock Garrison in 1680. Practising medicine, 1682-85. Granted 400 acres in 1684 for
transporting eight persons. In 1685 he either died or
disappeared, and the personal property in the house

he formerly lived in was seized to pay quit rents, levies, etc.

(Rappahannock Co. Records; Bruce: Institutional History of Va.)

TANKERLEY, DR. ————:
Paid for medical services by Vestry of Christ Church, Middlesex Co., 1696.
(Vestry Book, Christ Church.)

TAYLOR, DR. FRANCIS:
Born about 1631. Practising in Surry Co., 1673-83.
(Surry Co. Records.)

TAYLOR, JAMES:
Chirurgeon. His wife sued him for a separation in 1653, on grounds of adultery.
(Surry Co. Records.)

THORNBURY, WILLIAM:
Collected a fee for medical services in Rappahannock Co. in 1686.
(Rappahannock Co. Records.)

THRUSTON, DR. EDWARD:
Born Jan. 1638/9, son of John Thruston, Chamberlain of Bristol, Eng. Came to Va. in 1666, and settled at Martin's Hundred. Returned to England in 1671, but was again living in Va., in Norfolk Co., in 1717.
(Encyc. of Va. Biog.)

TICKNER, STEPHEN:
Chirurgeon. Mentioned in 1657, when he signed a contract agreeing to take Charles Clay as his apprentice and teach him physic and chirurgery.
(Surry Co. Records.)

TILLEY, DR. ————— :
 Mentioned, 1680.
 (York Co. Records.)

TILNEY, JOHN:
 His passage to Va. was paid for, before 1639, by Dr.
 John Holloway. In 1643 Dr. Holloway bequeathed
 him "all my Phisick and Chirurgery wth the chest
 Instruments, and Lancetts, all my phisicall and chi-
 rurgicall bookes Latin & English one small brasse
 morter and Pestle, one Cesterne . . ."
 (Northampton Co. Records.)

TOTON, DR. JOHN:
 Born about 1639. Lived at James City, but had a
 large practice in York Co. between 1678 and 1695.
 He was paid from the public funds in 1684 for curing
 a wounded soldier at James River Garrison.
 (York Co. Records; Journals House of Burgesses.)

TOWNSHEND (TOWNSEND), CAPTAIN RICHARD:
 Born 1606 or 1607. Came to Va. in 1620 as medical
 apprentice to Dr. Pott. Member House of Burgesses
 in 1628. Justice of York Co. in 1633, and presiding
 Justice in 1646. Member of the Council, 1636/7, and
 again from 1642 until 1646. Burgess again in 1642.
 Made frequent visits to England, where he is said to
 have been well connected. Owned a good deal of land
 in York Co. Died before 1650, leaving two sons,
 Francis and Robert.
 (Minutes of Council & General Court; Va. Mag. of
 Hist. & Biog., v. 9.)

TOWNSEND, DR. WILLIAM:
Practised in York Co. between 1678 and 1690.
(York Co. Records.)

TRACY, SAMUEL:
Probably a chirurgeon.   Mentioned as practising in
York Co. in 1661.
(York Co. Records.)

TUBB, DR. JAMES:
Lived in Charles City Co.   Mentioned, 1684-90.
(Henrico Co. and York Co. Records; Va. Mag. of
Hist. & Biog., v. 26.)

TURPIN, MICHAEL:
Probably a chirurgeon.   Mentioned, 1691.
(Henrico Co. Records.)

WAKE, RICHARD:
Chirurgeon, probably on the Ship *Elizabeth* of Lon-
don.   Was in Va. in 1625, and his inventory, taken in
Lower Norfolk Co., is dated Dec. 13, 1648.
(Minutes of Council & General Court; old MSS. in
the Richmond Academy of Medicine Library, Miller
Collection).

WALDRON, DR. HENRY:
Practised in Northampton Co., 1642-44, and in York
Co. 1646-57.   Died in Nov. 1657, leaving his "library
of bookes . . . with my chests of physicall meanes . . ."
to Dr. Robert Ellyson.
(Northampton & York Co. Records.)

WALE, GEORGE:
Probably a chirurgeon.   Practised in York Co. be-

tween 1657-62. Went to England in 1662, and probably remained there.
(York Co. Records.)

WALKER, DR. ————:
Mentioned, 1650.
(Va. Mag. of Hist. & Biog., v. 17.)

WALKER, DR. ————:
Mentioned, 1699.
(Neill: Va. Carolorum.)

WALLIS, DR. THOMAS:
Lived in Warwick River Co. Mentioned, 1647.
(York Co. Records.)

WALTER, MAXFIELD:
Ship surgeon. Bought land in Rappahannock Co. in 1675.
(Rappahannock Co. Records.)

WALTERS, RICHARD:
Ship surgeon, 1692.
(Va. Mag. of Hist. & Biog., v. 3.)

WARMAN, DR. STEPHEN:
Mentioned, 1663.
(Rappahannock Co. Records.)

WATER, DR. ROGER:
Practised in Rappahannock Co. and died there in 1685.
(Rappahannock Co. Records.)

WATKINS, DR. THOMAS:
Practising in York Co. in 1671, 1679, 1680.
(York Co. Records.)

WATKINSON, DR. THOMAS:
Practised in 1670-87. Was granted 200 acres in York
Co. in 1680. Died 1687.
(York Co. Records.)

WATSON, RALPH:
Chirurgeon. Died in 1645, leaving a fairly large
library.
(York Co. Records.)

WHITAKER, DR. WALTER:
Born about 1638. Practised in Middlesex Co. where
he was a Justice in 1673, 1681 and 1687, and High
Sheriff in 1685. Was called both "Captain" and
"Doctor." Died July 27, 1692. Member of the ves-
try of Christ Church in 1671.
(Minutes of Council & General Court; Executive
Journals, Council of Colonial Va.; Va. Mag. of Hist.
& Biog., v. 2, 8, 22; Vestry Book, Christ Church.)

WHITING, DR. HENRY:
Mentioned in Gloucester Co. in 1671 and York Co. in
1679. Justice of Gloucester Co., 1680; also Major
of Militia. Member of Council, 1691; Treasurer of
the Colony, 1692/3.
(Va. Mag. of Hist. & Biog., v. 18.)

WILKINSON, WILL:
Chirurgeon. Came to Va. in 1607.
(Smith: General History.)

WILLIAMS, JOHN:
Dutch chirurgeon, who was an indentured servant in
Va. in 1640. He took part in a plot to escape to the

"Dutch plantation," and as punishment was ordered to serve the colony for seven years.
(Minutes of Council & General Court.)

WILLIAMS, ROBERT:
Ship surgeon, 1651.
(Neill: Va. Carolorum.)

WILLIAMSON, DR. JAMES:
Justice of Lancaster Co. in 1652. John Hammond's "Leah and Rachel" was dedicated to him. Died before 1656.
(Encyc. Va. Biog.; Wm. & Mary Quart., v. 20; Force: Tracts, "Leah and Rachel".)

WILLIAMSON, DR. ROBERT:
Lived in Isle of Wight County. Member House of Burgesses in 1663 and 1666. Patented 3,850 acres on Blackwater Swamp, and had other grants of land. His will was dated Feb. 16, 1669.
(Va. Mag. of Hist. & Biog., v. 25.)

WILLOUGHBY, DR. HENRY:
Owned land in Rappahannock Co., and died there Nov. 28, 1685, leaving a library of 200 books.
(Rappahannock Co. Records.)

WILSON, JEOFFREY:
Probably a chirurgeon. Practised in York Co., 1658-61.
(York Co. Records.)

WINTERS (WINTER), DR. ANDREW:
Died in 1678, leaving a very small estate in York Co.
(York Co. Records.)

WOODSON, JOHN:
 "Phesition." Came to Virginia in 1619 with his wife, Sarah.
 (Va. Mag. of Hist. & Biog., v. 27.)

WOTTON (WOOTTON), THOMAS:
 Chirurgeon. Came to Va. in 1607, and was the first Surgeon-General of the colony. He was probably the same Thomas Wotton who went on a voyage to the East Indies in 1635 with Sir William Curteen, and died in 1638.
 (Smith: General History; Va. Mag. of Hist. & Biog., v. 22.)

WYTHE, DR. JOHN:
 Lived in Warwick Co. in 1704.
 (Wm. & Mary Quart., v. 4.)

BIBLIOGRAPHY

ANDERSON, L. B. Brief Biographies. Richmond, 1889.

BAAS, J. H. Outlines of the History of Medicine and the Medical Profession. Translated by Handerson.

BALL, J. M. The Sack-'Em-Up Men. London, 1928.

BALLAGH, JAMES C. White Servitude in the Colony of Virginia. Johns Hopkins University Studies, 13th Series, 1895.

BARTON, R. T. Reports by Sir John Randolph and Edward Barradall of Decisions of the General Court of Virginia. Introduction. 2 vols. Boston, 1909.

BERENGER-FERAUD, L. J. B. Traite Theorique et Clinique de la Fievre Jaune.

BEVERLEY, ROBERT. The History of Virginia. Reprint. Richmond, 1855.

BLOOMBAUGH, C. C. Roman and Greek Fees. Johns Hopkins Hosp. Bull. Baltimore, 1898, vol. IX.

BROWN, ALEXANDER. The First Republic in America. New York, 1898.
     The Genesis of the United States. 2 vols. New York, 1897.

BRUCE, PHILIP ALEXANDER. Economic History of Virginia in the Seventeenth Century. 2 vols. New York, 1896.
     Institutional History of Virginia in the Seventeenth Century. 2 vols. New York, 1910.
     Social Life of Virginia in the Seventeenth Century. Richmond, 1907.

BULLOCK, WILLIAM. Virginia impartially examined. London, 1649.

BURK, JOHN. The History of Virginia. 4 vols. Peters-burg, 1804.

BURR, GEORGE L. Narratives of the Witchcraft Cases, 1648-1706. New York, 1914.

BYRD, WILLIAM, SR. Letters of. Printed in the Va. Mag. of Hist. and Biog.

BYRD, WILLIAM, II. Writings. Edited by John Spencer Bassett. New York, 1901.

CALENDAR OF STATE PAPERS, COLONIAL SERIES. Edited by W. Noel Sainsbury. London, 1860.

CALENDAR OF VIRGINIA STATE PAPERS. 1 vol., 1652-1781. Edited by William P. Palmer. Richmond, 1875.

CAMPBELL, CHARLES. History of the Colony and Ancient Dominion of Virginia. Philadelphia, 1860.

CHASTELLUX, MARQUIS DE. Travels through North America, in the years 1780-81-82. New York, 1828.

CLAYTON, JOHN. A Letter from Mr. John Clayton, Rector of Crofton at Wakefield in Yorkshire to the Royal Society. Printed in Force: Tracts, vol. 3.

COLLECTIONS OF THE VIRGINIA HISTORICAL SOCIETY. New series. Edited by R. A. Brock.

COLONIAL RECORDS OF VIRGINIA. Senate Document. Printed from transcripts by McDonald and De Jar-nette of papers in the British Public Record Office. Richmond, 1874.

COUNTY RECORDS FOR THE SEVENTEENTH CENTURY. Certified copies in the Virginia State Library.

Elizabeth City.	1684-99.
Henrico.	1677-1700.
Northampton.	1632-45.
Northumberland.	1663.

Rappahannock.	1654-92.
Richmond.	1692-94.
Surry.	1645-86.
York.	1633-1702.

CRIDLIN, W. B. A History of Colonial Virginia. 1923.

DAVIS, JOHN STAIGE. President's Address before the Medical Society of Virginia, 1923.

DILLER, THEODORE. Pioneer Medicine in Western Pennsylvania.

DOYLE, J. A. English Colonies in America. New York, 1889.

EARLE, ALICE M. Two Centuries of Costume in America.

ENCYCLOPEDIA OF VIRGINIA BIOGRAPHY. Edited by Lyon G. Tyler, 1915.

FISKE, JOHN. Old Virginia and her Neighbors. 1897.

FITZHUGH, WILLIAM. Letters of. Printed in Va. Mag. of Hist. and Biog.

FORCE, PETER. Tracts and Other Papers. 4 vols. Washington, 1844.

GARRISON, FIELDING. History of Medicine. 1924.

GATFORD, LIONEL. Publicke Good without Private Interest. London, 1657.

GLOVER, THOMAS. Account of Virginia. Reprinted from the Philosophical Transactions of the Royal Society, June 20, 1676. Oxford, 1904.

GOODWIN, E. L. The Colonial Church in Virginia. Milwaukee, 1927.

GREER, GEORGE C. Early Virginia Immigrants, 1623-66. Richmond, 1912.

GROOME, H. C. Fauquier during the Proprietorship. Richmond, 1927.

HAGGARD, H. W. Devils, Drugs and Doctors. New York, 1929.

HAKLUYT, RICHARD. Collection of Early Voyages, Travels and Discoveries of the English Nation. London, 1809-12.

HAMMOND, JOHN. Leah and Rachel. London, 1656. Reprinted in Force: Tracts, vol. 3.

HAMOR, RALPH. A True Discourse of the Present State of Virginia. London, 1615. Reprint.

HARRIOT, THOMAS. A Briefe and True Report of the New Found Land of Virginia. 1588.

HARPERS MAGAZINE, Jan. 1886.

HARTWELL, CHILTON AND BLAIR. An Account of the Present State and Government of Virginia. London, 1727. Reprinted in Massachusetts Historical Society Collections, First Series, vol. 5.

HAYDEN, HORACE E. Virginia Genealogies.

HENING, WILLIAM WALLER. The Statutes at Large. Vols. 1, 2, 3. New York, 1823.

HUILLARD-BREHALLES. Diplomatic History of Frederick II.

INGLE, ED. Annals of Medical History, vol. v, 1924.

JAMES, EDWARD W. Lower Norfolk County Virginia Antiquary. 5 vols.

JEFFERSON, THOMAS. Notes on Virginia.

JONES, HUGH. The Present State of Virginia. London, 1724. Reprinted, New York, 1865.

KELLY, HOWARD, AND WALTER BURRAGE. Dictionary of
American Medical Biography. New York, 1928.

LANCET. London. 1915. Article on Sixteenth and Seven-
teenth Century Fees.
LEDERER, JOHN. Discoveries 1669-1670. Edited by
H. A. Ratterman. Cincinnati, 1879.
LONDON MAGAZINE, 1745.

MCCORMAC, E. I. White Servitude in Maryland, 1634-
1820. Johns Hopkins University Studies, Series 22.
MCILWAINE, H. R. Executive Journals of the Council of
Colonial Virginia. 3 vols. Richmond, 1925.
    Journals of the House of Burgesses of Virginia.
Vols. 1619-1658/9; 1659/60-1693; 1693-1701.
    Minutes of the Council and General Court of Colo-
nial Virginia, 1622-32; 1670-76. With notes and
Excerpts from Original Council and General Court
Records into 1683, now lost. Richmond, 1924.
MEADE, BISHOP WILLIAM. Old Churches, Ministers and
Families of Virginia. Philadelphia, 1857.

NEILL, EDWARD D. The English Colonization of America
During the Seventeenth Century. London, 1871.
    History of the Virginia Company of London.
Albany, 1869.
    Virginia Carolorum. Albany, 1886.
    Virginia Vetusta. Albany, 1885.
NEW ENGLAND HISTORICAL AND GENEALOGICAL REGIS-
TER, 1888. vol. XLII.

OLDMIXON, JOHN. The British Empire in America. London, 1741.

Packard, F. R. History of Medicine in the United States. Philadelphia, 1901.

Parish Records:

Vestry Book and Register of Christ Church, Middlesex County, Virginia. Edited by C. G. Chamberlayne.

Annals of Henrico Parish and History of St. John's Church. Edited by J. S. Moore.

Vestry Book of Saint Peter's, New Kent County, Virginia. Published by the Society of the Colonial Dames in the State of Virginia.

(Note: Other published parish records do not date farther back than the Eighteenth Century.)

Percy, George. Discourse. Printed in Arber's introduction to the Works of Captain John Smith; also in Brown: Genesis, and Purchas: Pilgrimes.

Phillips, Ulrich Bonnell. Life and Labor in the Old South. 1929.

Purchas, Samuel. Pilgrimes. London, 1625-26. 5 vols.
Pilgrimage. London, 1617.

Rogers, J. E. T. History of Agriculture and Prices in England. Oxford, 1887.

Royal Society, Philosophical Transactions of the. 1690-94.

Smith, Captain John. Works, 1608-1631. Edited by Edward Arber. Birmingham, 1884. (Includes the General Historie of Virginia.)

Spelman, Henry. Relation of Virginia, 1609. London, 1872.

SQUIRES, W. H. T. The Days of Yester-Year in Colony and Commonwealth. Portsmouth, 1928.

STANARD, MARY NEWTON. Colonial Virginia, Its People and Customs. Philadelphia and London, 1917.
    The Story of Virginia's First Century. Philadelphia, 1928.

STITH, WILLIAM. The History of the First Discovery and Settlement of Virginia. Williamsburg, 1747. Reprinted, New York, 1865.

STRACHEY, WILLIAM. The Historie of Travaile into Virginia Britannia. (Written 1616-18.) Printed from the original manuscript in the British Museum, London, 1849.

THACHER, JAMES. American Medical Biography. 2 vols. Boston, 1828.

TONER, J. M. Contributions to the Annals of Medical Progress and Medical Education in the United States, 1874.

TORRENCE, WILLIAM CLAYTON. A Trial Bibliography of Colonial Virginia. Richmond, 1908.

TYLER, LYON G. Cradle of the Republic. Richmond, 1900.

U. S. CENSUS. 1910. Vol. 3.

VAUGHAN, W. T. An Epidemiologic Study.

VIRGINIA COMPANY OF LONDON, RECORDS OF THE. The Court Book. Edited by S. M. Kingsbury. Vols. 1, 2. Washington, 1906.

VIRGINIA HISTORICAL MAGAZINE. Edited by Jefferson Maxwell. 1 vol. Richmond, 1891-92.

Virginia Historical Register. Edited by William Maxwell. 6 vols. 1848-54. Richmond.

Virginia Magazine of History and Biography. Published Quarterly by the Virginia Historical Society. 1894-1929.

Virginia Richly and Truly Valued. 1650. Reprinted in Force: Tracts, v. 3.

Walsh, J. J. Medical Fees down the Ages. Internat. Clin. Phil. 1910, v. IV.

Fee Book of a Seventeenth Century Irish Physician. N. Y. Med. Journal, 1912, v. XCVI.

History of Medicine in New York, 5 vols. New York, 1919.

Wertenbaker, Thomas Jefferson. Planters of Colonial Virginia. Princeton, 1922.

Virginia under the Stuarts. Princeton, 1913.

William and Mary College Quarterly. 1892-1919. Second series, 1921-1929.

Wingfield, Edward Maria. Discourse of Virginia. Printed from the original manuscript in the Lambeth Library. Boston, 1859. (Also in Arber's Introduction to Works of Captain John Smith.)

Wise, Jennings C. Ye Kingdome of Accawmacke, or the Eastern Shore of Virginia in the Seventeenth Century. Richmond, 1911.

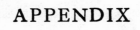

APPENDIX

APPENDIX

A

Alsine Spergula latifolia reptans.
  Becabungae folio.
Althaea lutea Pimpinellae majoris folio, floribus parvis,
    seminibus rostratis.   Folia hujus plantae pediculis in-
    sident.
Althaea magna Aceris folio, cortice Cannabino, floribus
    parvis semina rotatim in summitate caulium, singula
    singulis cuticulis rostratis, cooperta ferens.
Althaea magna quinquecapsularis, cortice Cannabino, foliis
    integris subtus albicantibus, floribus magnis ex fundo
    saturatè rubro albis.
Alth. magna quinquecapsularis cortice Cannabino, foliis
    Malvarum modo divisis, subtus, viridibus.
Ambrosia inodora foliis non divisis.
  gigantea inodora foliis asperis trifidis.
Anchusa lutea minor, quam Indi Paccoon vocant seipsos ea
    pingentes.
Anemone latifolia sylvestris alba.
Apocynum erectum non ramosum folio subrotundo, umbellis
    florum rubris.
Apoc. erect. non ramos. latiore folio, umbellis florum albi-
    cantibus.
Apoc. erect. minus, umbellâ florum candida.

---

*From Ray's Historia Plantarum, p. 1926.

Apoc. erect. non ram. Asclepiadis folio, umbellis florum
    rubentibus.
Apoc. minus non lactescens, caule & foliis hirsutis, floribus
    saturatè luteis.
Apoc. erect. non ram. Roris marini foliis umbellis florum
    candidis.
Apoc. petraeum ramosum Salicis folio.
Apoc. scandens, capsulis brevibus spinis asperis.
Apoc. scand. capsulis alatis.
Apoc. scand. capsulis planis.
    Haec omnia siliquas ferunt tumentes.
Apoc. erect. ramosum, caule rubente, foliis oblongis parvis,
    siliquis (ex flosculis albis) tenuissimis, binatim ad ex-
    tremitates conjunctis.
Arisarum triphyllum, pene viridi.
Aris. triph. minus, pene atro-rubente.
Aris. Dracontii foliis pene longo acuminato.
Arum aquaticum, foliis in acumen desinentibus, fructu viridi.
Arum fluitans, pene nudo.

C

Carduus Jaceoides purp. foliis subtus incanis, capite viscoso.
Caryophyllata flore semper albo.
Castanea pumila racemoso fructu parvo, in singulis capsulis
    echinatis unico, The Chinquapin. Autor descriptionis
    Carolinae ex hac nuce Chocolatam fieri refert non
    multò inferiorem ei quae ex Cacao fit.
Centaurium minus caule quadrato alato, flore carneo amplo,
    umbilico luteo.
Centaurium luteum Ascyroides.
Clematis purpurea repens petalis florum coriaceis.

Clem. erecta, humilis non ramosa, foliis subrotundis, flore
unico ochroleuco.
Cochlearia flore majori In locis udis a salsis procul remotis.
Conyza coerulea acris Americana.
Cucumis fructu minimo viridi, ad maturitatem perducto
nigricante.   Fructus Bryoniae albae baccâ non multo
major est, cujus primo aspectu speciem esse putaveram.

D
Dens caninus flore luteo.
Digitalis flore pallido transparenti, foliis & caule molli hir-
sutie imbutis.
Digit. rubra minor, labiis florum patulis, foliis parvis angustis.
Digit. lutea elatior Jaceae nigrae foliis. lutea altera, foliis
tenuius dissectis thecis florum foliaceis. parva comis
coccineis.

E
Eryngium campestre Yuccae foliis, spinis tenellis hinc inde
marginibus appositis.
Euonymus capsulis eleganter bullatis.

F
Filix mas foliis integris auriculatis.
    mas rachi seu nervo medio alato.
    foemina foliis per margines pulverulentis, seminibus fim-
    briatis.
Fumaria siliquosa lutea.
    Siliquosa altera grumosa radice, floribus gemellis ad
    labia conjunctis.

Fungus (ex stercore equino) capillaceus capitulo rorido, nigro punctulo in summitate notato. Ex recenti fimo noctu exoritur cauliculis erectis, vix digitum longis, capillorum instar tenuibus nec minus densis seu confertis. Singuli Cauliculi parvulo globulo aqueo coronantur, qui in summa sui parte macula parva nigra Limacis oculo simili insignitur.

G

Gentianae affinis foliis glabris serratis, floribus Ranae referentibus.
Gladiolus caeruleus hexapetalos, caule etiam gladiato.
Gratiola foliis latioribus serratis.

H

Hedera trifolia Canadensis foliis sinuatis.
Helleborine flore rotundo luteo, purpureis venis striato.
　The Mockasine flower.
Helxine latè scandens seminibus majoribus.
Helxine frutescens Bryoniae nigrae foliis, capsulis triquetris amplis Pergamenis.
Hieracium fruticosum latifolium foliis punctulis & venis sanguineis notatis.
Hyacinthus Occidentalis flore pallidè coeruleo.
Hypericum parvum caule quadrato seu Ascyron minimum.
Hyper. pumilum semper virens caule compresso ligneo; ad bina latera alato, flore luteo tetrapetalo, seu Crux S. Andreae.
Hyper. frutescens luteum Phillyrrheae foliis.

J

Jacea non ramosa tuberosa radice, foliis plurimis rigidis perangustis, flores ferens multos parvos rubentes acaules in spica ad caulem sessiles.

Jac. non ram. tub. rad. foliis latioribus flores ferens pauciores, majores, squamis hiantibus armatos & pediculis curtis insidentes.

Jacobaea lanata foliis brevibus subrotundis, lanata altera foliis longis angustis.

Jasminum arboreum foliis amplis, oblongis, supernè virentibus, subtus leni canitie pubescentibus, flores albos in quatuor lacinias longas angustas ad umbilicum usque partitos racematim ferens.

Iris aculeata baccifera arborea minùs ferax.

Iris coerulea latifolia & angustifolia.

Chamae-Iris verna odoratissima, latifolia coerulea repens.

L

Pseudo-Lathyrus luteus glaber, siliquis tumentibus, duplicem seminum seriem continentibus.

Pseudo-Lath. lut. hirsutus siliq. tument. continentibus duplicem seriem seminum.

Laurus Tinus floribus albidis eleganter bullatis. Flos nondum apertus pyxidi S. M. Magdalenae (ut nonnunquam pictam vidi) similis est.

Lilio-narcissus humilis albus.

Lilium S. Martagnon floribus reflexis ex luteo rubentibus, purpureis maculis eleganter notatis.

Lilium S. Martagnon pusillum florib. minutissimis herbaceis. Caulem habet vix dodrantalem, verticillo foliorum uni-

co cinctum, cujus summitas quatuor floribus reflexis
Solani lignosi floribus magnitudine haud aequalibus,
pediculis parvis insidentibus coronantur.

Lilium Squillae foliis, denticellis parvis ad margines serratis.   Caule est alto, nudo, ad cujus summitatem prodeunt flores in spica sessiles, petalis paene ad imum
(ut loqui amant feciales) quasi erasis; staminibus sex
(si non malè memini) purpuro-coeruleis, mole sua
aliquantulum depressis.   Flos quamvis aspectu non admodum pulcher sit pergratum habet odorem.   Radicem habet imbricatam instar Lilii, folia crassa admodum & succulenta, non tamen Sempervivi species est.

Lonchitis maxima foliis planis i. e. non dentatis, nec pulverulentis maculis notatis, uno in cespite foliorum unicum protrudens caulem foliis angustioribus, pulverem
seu semina in membranulis quasi in capsulis ferentibus
compositum.

Lonchitis major Polydodii facie.   Haec atque etiam vulgaris simili modo florida est.

Lychnis plumaria alba, foliis ad geniculum quatuor cruciatim positis, thecis florum tumentibus.

Lysimachia lutea minor, foliis & floribus purpureo punctatis.

Lysimachia siliquosa lutea minor.

M

Melissa elatior foliis magnis dentatis glabris, ad geniculum
binis: flores odoratos luteos patulos stamina bina
quasi cornua protrudentibus in summitate caulium racematim ferens.

Mercurialis tricoccos hermaphroditica, s. ad foliorum juncturas ex foliolis cristatis Julifera simul ac fructum
ferens.

Muscus erectus densè complicatus Cupressi foliis major &
  minor. In rupe quadam prope Sabinas foliis Cupressi.
Myrrhis minor procumbens, seu potius Cerefolium.

N

Nux vesicaria Virginiana Park.

O

Orchis palmata elegans lutea cum longis calcaribus luteis,
  palmata lutea minor nullis calcaribus. Hermaphroditica, flore minore, calcare longiore.
Origanum floribus amplis luteis, purpureo maculatis, cujus
  caulis sub quovis verticillo decem vel duodecimo foliis
  est circumcinctus.
Orig. cujus ramorum summitates floribus dilutè rubris in
  verticillos congestis coronantur.
Orig. foliis ad summitatem caulium canis, floribus multis
  pallidè coeruleis in cymis ramorum densè stipatis.
Ornithogalum luteum parvum foliis gramineis hirsutis.
Orobanche radice dentata caule & flore albo. Flos ejus
  quem unicum in uno caule Goodyeri Orobanches
  similis est sed major. Conceptaculi seminalis venter
  seu pars protuberans non rotunda est sed canaliculata.

P

Pepo fructu parvo compresso.
Phalangium ramosum floribus albis, ad fundum viridibus.
Phalangium album non ramosum floribus albis ad caulem
  spicatim sessilibus.
Phyllitis parva saxatilis per summitates folii prolifera.

Pisum spontaneum purpureum.
Plantago aquatica latiore folio.
Polygala seu Flos ambarvalis floribus luteis in caput ob-
longum congestis.
Polyg. rubra spicâ parvâ compacta.
Polygala spicata rubra major foliis & caulibus coerulescen-
tibus.
Pol. quadrifolia S. cruciata floribus ex viridi rubentibus, in
globum compactis.
Pol. quadrif. minor spica parva rubente.
Polygonatum ramosum capsulâ prismaticâ, ramosum per-
foliatum flore ochroleuco capsula trigonâ.
Polypodium parvum foliis minutim serratis.
Polypodium minus alterum Scolopendriae facie.
Potamogiton Virginianum.

Q

Quercus variae species, 1. Pumila. 2. Alba. 3. Rubra.
4. Hispanica. 5. Castaneae folio. 6. Lini aut Salicis
foliis. 7. Fruticosa. Harum primam in Historia,
quintam in Appendice meminimus.

R

Ranunculus Thalictri folio, radice grumosa; Anemone sylv.
Rapuntum minimum glabrum. In uliginosis minùs glabrum
flore pallidiorè.
Rhamnus Prunifolius fructu nigro, ossiculo compresso. The
Black Haw.
Rhus ramis ex stipite pullulantibus glabris. Hujus truncus
carpi crassitiem nunquam superat, pollicis raro exce-

dit. Baccae sapore sunt subsalso cum pungenti illo
acore qui in Tamarindis sentitur mixto.
Rubia parva foliolis ad geniculum unumquodque binis, flore
coeruleo fistuloso.
Rub parva latifolia foliis ad genic. binis, flore rubente.

S

Sanicula seu Auricula ursi Cyclamini flore.
Saxifraga petraea Alsinefolia.
Sedum saxatile parvum, caule gracili aphyllo, floribus
rubentibus.
Solanum verticillatum latifolium molle, floribus obsoletè
rubris, baccis luteis.
Sol. verticill. angustiore folio, flore ochroleuco.
Sol. triphyllum flo. tripetalo, atro-purpureo, in foliorum
sinu absque pediculo sessili.
Staphis agria fol. dilutè viridibus.
Stramonium fundo floris coeruleo, pomis longioribus spinis
armatis.

T

Trichomanes major foliis longis auriculatis.

U

Valeriana Graeca seu Valeriana coerulea minor.
Veronica pratensis Serpyllifolia.
Viola tricolor nudo caule, foliis tenuius dissectis.
Viola alabastrites pentaphyllea, Cochleariae sapore, Nas-
turtii species.
Urtica urens major seminibus rotundis, compressis locula-
mentis viridibus inclusis & in caulis summitate racema-
tim dispositis.

Inter semina ad me è Virginia transmissa, Anno 1687. ad
    eodem D. Banister, nonnulla invenio quorum nomina
    in hoc Catalogo non habentur, v. g.
Erigeron (frutex marit.)   Halimi folio: Senecio arbores-
    cens Atriplicis folio.
Eryngium Plinii Portulacae foliis à D. Spragge acceptum.
Euonymus (ni malè memini) Pyracanthae foliis.
Lysimachia lutea corniculata maritima.
Cynoglossum coeruleum Buglossi foliis.
Senae spuriae tres species quarum una siliquis est hirsutis à
    D. Spragge acceptae.   Duae à me satae germinârunt
    & plantas produxerunt, quae duae species Paiomirio-
    bae à Pisone descriptae esse videbantur.
Pistacia nigra Coryli folio D. Spragge.
Ulmus fructu Lupulino.
Ricinus parvus Urticae folio.
Convolvulus bicapsularis seminibus pappo alatis.
Phalangium spicatum flosculo Arbuteo bullato aureo.
Lithospermum floribus rostratis.
Ricinus frutescens Fici foliis.
Gramen marinum echinatum.   Hujus semina etiam à D.
    Spragge accepi, quae hac aestate in horto sata germin-
    arunt, sed nondum ad frugem pervenerunt.

INDEX

Index

Abram, Dr. Thomas, 260.
Accidents, a cause of high mortality, 42.
Accounts. *See* Fees.
Acmunist (alchemist?), 107.
Actuarius, 141.
Addams, Dr. William, 260.
Agriculture, interest of physicians in, 233.
Ague, 11, 39, 51, 52, 53, 68, 111, 219.
Air, influence on health, 218.
Albertus Magnus, 95.
Alchemy, 119.
Alkermes, Confectio, 118.
Allcock, Thomas, 129.
Allen, Dr. Nathaniell, 260.
Allenagra, red earth, 104.
Allerton, Isaac, 189.
Allin, Dr., 260.
Allington, Giles, 167.
Allum-water, 101.
Aloes, 114.
Alum, 108, 114; rock, plain, 100; red, carthagena, roach, Romish, 104.
Amenorrhoea, black snake root used to cure, 109.
Ammonia, aromatic spirits of, 114, 115.
Amputation, 120, 144, 145.
Anatomy, 79, 120, 121, 231.
Anderson, William, 221.
Andrews, Dr. Henry, 91, 260.
Andros, Governor, 62.
Anemia, use of iron in, 121.
Anesthesia, 144.
Annis, John, 92.
Anthony, Francis, subscriber to the London Company, 5.
Antilles, yellow fever in the, 72, 73, 74.
Antimony, 113, 122.
Antisepsis, 164.
Ants, 105.

Apothecaries, 5, 8, 9, 21, 24, 25, 31, 64, 110, 111, 115, 116, 133.
Appendicitis, 125.
Apple, thorny, of Peru, 112.
Applications, external, 118.
Apprenticeship, 21, 24, 31, 80, 86, 87, 88, 96, 97, 164, 185.
Archer, Gabriel, 34, 58, 70.
Arderne, John, 135, 236.
Argoll, Sir Samuel, 101.
Arnold, Dr., 157, 260.
Arundale, William, 166.
Aselli, Gasparo, 121.
Asepsis, 144.
Astringents, 117, 118.
Astrology, 119; Christian, 255.
Asylum, for the insane, at Williamsburg, 128.
Austin, Robert, 184.
Autopsies, 79, 201, 202.
Avicenna, 79, 141.
Aylett, Mr. Thomas, 260.

Back Street, Dr. Pott's house on, 12, 20.
Bacon, Nathaniel, 156; Rebellion of, 24, 42, 112, 194; the elder, 177.
Baglivi, George, 122.
Bagnall, Anthony, chirurgeon, 9, 10, 210, 261.
Baker, Sir George, 66.
Ball, J. M., 201.
Baltimore, Lord, 23; Lady, 132.
Banbury, Sarah, lying-in of, 157.
Banister, Rev. John, 215, 216, 261, 309.
Bankes, Dr. William, 196, 233, 261.
Banton, Dr., 261.
Barbadoes, 37, 114, 126, 220; Distemper, 72.
Barbeirac, Charles, 80.
Barbers, 6, 123, 138, 144, 207; College, 80.

[321]

Medicine & Society In America

An Arno Press/New York Times Collection

Alcott, William A. **The Physiology of Marriage.** 1866. New Introduction by Charles E. Rosenberg.

Beard, George M. **American Nervousness:** Its Causes and Conse-
quences. 1881. New Introduction by Charles E. Rosenberg.

Beard, George M. **Sexual Neurasthenia.** 5th edition. 1898.

Beecher, Catharine E. **Letters to the People on Health and Happiness.** 1855.

Blackwell, Elizabeth. **Essays in Medical Sociology.** 1902. Two
volumes in one.

Blanton, Wyndham B. **Medicine in Virginia in the Seventeenth
Century.** 1930.

Bowditch, Henry I. **Public Hygiene in America.** 1877.

Bowditch, N[athaniel] I. **A History of the Massachusetts General
Hospital:** To August 5, 1851. 2nd edition. 1872.

Brill, A. A. **Psychanalysis:** Its Theories and Practical Applica-
tion. 1913.

Cabot, Richard C. **Social Work:** Essays on the Meeting-Ground of
Doctor and Social Worker. 1919.

Cathell, D. W. **The Physician Himself and What He Should Add to
His Scientific Acquirements.** 2nd edition. 1882. New Introduction
by Charles E. Rosenberg.

The Cholera Bulletin. Conducted by an Association of Physicians.
Vol. I: Nos. 1–24. 1832. All published. New Introduction by
Charles E. Rosenberg.

Clarke, Edward H. **Sex in Education;** or, A Fair Chance for the
Girls. 1873.

Committee on the Costs of Medical Care. **Medical Care for the
American People:** The Final Report of The Committee on the
Costs of Medical Care, No. 28. [1932].

Currie, William. **An Historical Account of the Climates and Diseases of the United States of America.** 1792.

Davenport, Charles Benedict. **Heredity in Relation to Eugenics.**
1911. New Introduction by Charles E. Rosenberg.

Davis, Michael M. **Paying Your Sickness Bills.** 1931.

Disease and Society in Provincial Massachusetts: Collected Accounts, 1736–1939. 1972.

Earle, Pliny. **The Curability of Insanity:** A Series of Studies. 1887.

Falk, I. S., C. Rufus Rorem, and Martha D. Ring. **The Costs of
Medical Care:** A Summary of Investigations on The Economic
Aspects of the Prevention and Care of Illness, No. 27. 1933.

Faust, Bernhard C. **Catechism of Health:** For the Use of Schools,
and for Domestic Instruction. 1794.

Flexner, Abraham. **Medical Education in the United States and Canada:** A Report to The Carnegie Foundation for the Advancement of Teaching, Bulletin Number Four. 1910.

Gross, Samuel D. **Autobiography of Samuel D. Gross, M.D.,** with Sketches of His Contemporaries. Two volumes. 1887.

Hooker, Worthington. **Physician and Patient;** or, A Practical View of the Mutual Duties, Relations and Interests of the Medical Profession and the Community. 1849.

Howe, S. G. **On the Causes of Idiocy.** 1858.

Jackson, James. **A Memoir of James Jackson, Jr., M.D.** 1835.

Jennings, Samuel K. **The Married Lady's Companion, or Poor Man's Friend.** 2nd edition. 1808.

The Maternal Physician; a Treatise on the Nurture and Management of Infants, from the Birth until Two Years Old. 2nd edition. 1818. New Introduction by Charles E. Rosenberg.

Mathews, Joseph McDowell. **How to Succeed in the Practice of Medicine.** 1905.

McCready, Benjamin W. **On the Influences of Trades, Professions, and Occupations in the United States, in the Production of Disease.** 1943.

Mitchell, S. Weir. **Doctor and Patient.** 1888.

Nichols, T[homas] L. **Esoteric Anthropology:** The Mysteries of Man. [1853].

Origins of Public Health in America: Selected Essays, 1820–1855. 1972.

Osler, Sir William. **The Evolution of Modern Medicine.** 1922.

The Physician and Child-Rearing: Two Guides, 1809–1894. 1972.

Rosen, George. **The Specialization of Medicine:** with Particular Reference to Ophthalmology. 1944.

Royce, Samuel. **Deterioration and Race Education.** 1878.

Rush, Benjamin. **Medical Inquiries and Observations.** Four volumes in two. 4th edition. 1815.

Shattuck, Lemuel, Nathaniel P. Banks, Jr., and Jehiel Abbott. **Report of a General Plan for the Promotion of Public and Personal Health.** Massachusetts Sanitary Commission. 1850.

Smith, Stephen. **Doctor in Medicine** and Other Papers on Professional Subjects. 1872.

Still, Andrew T. **Autobiography of Andrew T. Still,** with a History of the Discovery and Development of the Science of Osteopathy. 1897.

Storer, Horatio Robinson. **The Causation, Course, and Treatment of Reflex Insanity in Women.** 1871.

Sydenstricker, Edgar. **Health and Environment.** 1933.

Thomson, Samuel. **A Narrative, of the Life and Medical Discoveries of Samuel Thomson.** 1822.

Ticknor, Caleb. **The Philosophy of Living;** or, The Way to Enjoy Life and Its Comforts. 1836.

U.S. Sanitary Commission. **The Sanitary Commission of the United States Army:** A Succinct Narrative of Its Works and Purposes. 1864.

White, William A. **The Principles of Mental Hygiene.** 1917.